"Dr. Chan's book is a thoughtful, comprehensive resource for the patient who has been diagnosed with breast cancer. He has been able to simplify, very succinctly, answers to the most complex questions raised by one facing this disease and its treatment. I would recommend this book, without hesitation, to breast cancer patients, who often feel lost in an abyss of complex medical information."

—LINNEA I. CHAP, MD,
Co-Director of the Revlon/UCLA Breast Center
and Associate Professor of Medicine
at UCLA/Geffen School of Medicine

"This wonderful book does exactly what it says: provides the real answers to the many important questions asked by our breast cancer patients, in a style that is accessible to all. The answers are concise, accurate, up-to-date, and eminently readable. They reflect the true nature of the author: a highly caring physician who has dedicated his life to battling this disease . . . which all of us aim to overcome in our lifetime."

—BRIAN LEYLAND-JONES, MD,
Director of the McGill Comprehensive Cancer Center
and Minda de Gunzburg Chair of Oncology
at McGill University in Montreal

"Dr. David Chan is a well-respected, well-trained, and inspirational medical oncologist. In his twenty years of clinical practice, breast cancer patients have asked him important questions about their disease and treatment. Dr. Chan has synthesized these questions and their answers in an easily read format. Most patients, in the whirlwind and tumult surrounding their breast cancer diagnosis, will find this book a useful tool for reflection and study. Their spouses and other loved ones are also likely to find David's book helpful."

—DOUGLAS W. BLAYNEY, MD,
Professor of Medicine
and Medical Director of the Comprehensive Cancer Center
at the University of Michigan Medical School

"A Google search of the Internet using the key term 'breast cancer' yields 21,700,000 hits. Using Medline to search only the peer-reviewed, medical research publications on the topic of breast cancer, one finds 138,188 papers in hundreds of different scientific journals. Imagine now a newly diagnosed patient (or their family members or helpful friends) with no medical background or knowledge of tumor biology, clinical research, epidemiology, pathology, or pharmacology, attempting to sift through this daunting amount of data in order to find answers to simple but critical clinical questions regarding their care. This situation creates severe anxiety and frustration for patients with the disease; moreover, some of the 'information' available on the Internet is not evidence-based, or worse yet, just plain wrong.

"Consequently, *Breast Cancer: Real Questions, Real Answers* meets a major unmet need for patients with breast cancer as it contains *the* most frequently asked questions about the disease, and presents concise (yet precise) practical, understandable, informative answers to these very common questions. This work is a 'must read' for patients as an entry point into the bewildering world of clinical decision making in management of breast cancer. The work is wonderfully illustrated providing an understandable framework for lessons on complex topics such as anatomy, pathology, genetics, diagnostic imaging, and even molecular biology. I will definitely plan to keep a copy of this book in the waiting room for patients in my clinic at UCLA."

—MARK D. PEGRAM, MD,
Associate Professor of Medicine at
UCLA/Geffen School of Medicine
and Director of the Women's Cancer Program at
the UCLA/Jonsson Comprehensive Cancer Center

"Dr. Chan is skillfully teaching the art as well as the science of breast cancer treatment in this excellent book. I am eagerly anticipating the French edition to benefit our patients and their loved ones."

—SYLVIE GIACCHETTI, MD,
Centre for Diseases of the Breast, Service d' Oncologie
at the Hospital Saint Louis in Paris

About the Author

Dr. David Chan is an oncologist in Redondo Beach, California, and is an instructor at the Revlon/UCLA Breast Center. He has treated over 2,500 breast cancer patients, and has written and lectured extensively on breast cancer over a twenty-year career. Dr. Chan received his medical degree at UCLA, and his oncology training at Stanford University. He is President of Cancer Care Associates, one of the leading oncology groups in Southern California. Dr. Chan also serves as Chairman of the Steering Committee of the Community/UCLA Oncology Network and is a Principal Investigator for the UCLA/Translational Oncology Institute. Dr. Chan and Cancer Care Associates are active in UCLA breast cancer clinical trials, striving to advance the treatment and cure of breast cancer.

BREAST CANCER

Real Questions, Real Answers

David Chan, MD

Illustrated by Eric F. Glassy, MD
Preface by John Glaspy, MD, MPH
Introduction by Frank Stockdale, MD, PhD

MARLOWE & COMPANY
NEW YORK

BREAST CANCER:
Real Questions, Real Answers

Published by
Marlowe & Company
An Imprint of Avalon Publishing Group Incorporated
245 West 17th Street • 11th floor
New York, NY 10011

AVALON
publishing group incorporated

Library of Congress Cataloging-in-Publication Data
Chan, David, 1953–
Breast cancer : real questions, real answers / David Chan ; illustrated by
Eric F. Glassy ; introduction by John Glaspy ; preface by Frank Stockdale.
p. cm.
Includes index.
ISBN 1-56924-314-X (pbk.)
1. Breast—Cancer. I. Title.
RC280.B8C473 2006
616.99'449—dc22
2005030690

ISBN-13: 978-1-56924-314-5

9 8 7 6 5 4 3 2

Designed by India Amos, Neuwirth and Associates, Inc.
Printed in the United States of America

For Suzy and Spencer

Contents

Illustrations and Tables

Preface

THE ULTIMATE QUESTION: What do women who have been diagnosed with breast cancer want from health care providers? My experience has been that the first thing they want from us is answers: clear, accurate, up-to-date, thorough but concise information they need to help them comprehend as much as possible what has happened and decide upon and implement a course of action that is right for them. To adequately meet this need, physicians treating breast cancer must be scientifically well-informed and clinically experienced, but also patient, compassionate, and forthright communicators, willing to devote sufficient time to providing the answers. This is a tall order, but an essential first step in securing the best possible outcome for each patient.

I have known Dr. David Chan since our medical school days, and have had the privilege of practicing academic oncology for twenty years in Southern California, where he is one of the most sought-after and respected clinical oncologists. Unflaggingly for all those years, Dave has been an integral and valued participant in our breast cancer program at UCLA, generously contributing his valuable time to our outpatient clinics and teaching conferences, helping us to fill the tall order for our patients, and sharing with the next generation of physicians his extensive knowledge and experience. Remarkably, in addition to providing his patients and ours with the answers they need, Dave has also been an active participant in our breast cancer research efforts, helping to generate new answers to questions for which we had none. Dave's work with UCLA has served as a model of what a relationship between a research center and an oncology practice can and should be.

No encounter between a patient and a physician is ever perfect and there is always the question unasked or the answer forgotten. That's the unfilled niche this book will fill. In a unique question and answer format, Dr. Chan provides clear, concise, and accurate answers to questions that he hears from patients on a daily basis. Women and their loved ones who are confronting breast cancer will find the information he provides empowering in preparing for or reflecting on their meetings with physicians. It will help them understand what has happened, what options exist and their rationale, what is known and unknown. Most important, it will support them in the process of making decisions that are right for them, choosing an approach they are comfortable will secure the best possible outcome. This book will help us fill the tall order.

JOHN GLASPY, MD, MPH
Professor of Medicine
Sanders Chair in Cancer Research
Director, Clinical Research Unit
Jonsson Comprehensive Cancer Center
UCLA School of Medicine
Los Angeles, California

Introduction

A S SOMEONE WHO has treated breast cancer for almost four decades, I have seen a marked shift from performing a mastectomy as the sole primary treatment of breast cancer to the current strategy of treating the entire patient. Breast surgery is now only one of a number of therapies used in a modern breast cancer treatment program. The advances in treatment over the last decade have been most impressive and I would like to highlight the major ones in this preface.

Today breast surgery is still an essential component of the treatment plan. There is, however, a very noticeable reduction in the number of mastectomies. The majority of women no longer need to lose their breast. In addition to surgical treatment, almost every newly diagnosed breast cancer patient receives some form of medical treatment such as hormonal therapy or chemotherapy to lower her chance of breast cancer relapse. This combination of reduced surgery and increased use of hormonal and chemotherapy has resulted in higher cure rates, reduced suffering, and better quality of life.

This last decade has been very important in virtually every aspect of breast cancer diagnosis and treatment, both for women with breast cancer and also for women who are at high risk of getting breast cancer. Even though analyses show a higher number of breast cancers now compared to ten years ago, the number of women dying today from the disease has significantly decreased as a direct result of improvements in diagnosing breast cancer earlier and in treating the disease.

It has been less than ten years since the first breast cancer susceptibility gene, BRCA1, was discovered and analyzed. This led to the discovery of a second gene, BRCA2, and the rapid development of a commercially available test permitting women in high-risk families to undergo genetic testing for risk assessment. Researchers studying these high-risk families have discovered that this genetic abnormality also increases a woman's chance of getting cancer of the ovary. In the past several years, more effective strategies for screening and prevention for high-risk women have been developed.

We have learned a lot about breast cancer risk reduction. We have known for decades that estrogen use could increase breast cancer risk but the degree of risk was often debated and difficult to estimate until recent studies were completed. It is now clearly established that postmenopausal use of estrogen increases a woman's chance of getting breast cancer and that with the addition of progesterone, the risk is increased even more. With recognition of important risk factors, the concept of breast cancer prevention has also emerged. We now know that taking Tamoxifen for five years can reduce the risk of breast cancer by almost 50 percent. Within just the past several years, we have also learned that another type of hormonal treatment, aromatase inhibitors, may be as effective in preventing breast cancer and possibly more so and with less side effects. These treatments offer very meaningful reductions in breast cancer risk and are now often used in higher risk women.

Imaging techniques for the early and more accurate diagnosis of breast cancer have improved considerably. It is common today to have mammograms scanned by computer-assisted analyzers to reduce reading errors. Additionally, the development of digital images can help make mammograms easier to read and lessens the chance of missing a cancer. Improvements in mammography have resulted in a decrease in the size of breast cancers diagnosed over the last decade and this will lead to higher cure rates. Recent developments in MRI analysis of the breast have added a new way to image the breast. MRI has the advantage of not using X-ray and is currently being used to screen high-risk women or women with dense breasts where mammograms are less helpful. Newer biopsy techniques allow most biopsies to be performed with a needle, reducing the need for surgical excisions of abnormalities seen on mammography or other imaging methods.

Advances in surgery have allowed many women to avoid an axillary dissection, a surgery that can lead to long-term discomfort and sometimes significant swelling of the arm. This important recent surgical advance is termed sentinel lymph node mapping, and replaces the standard axillary dissection. This surgery is just as accurate in assessing risk of cancer spread. Most breast cancer patients can now have sentinel lymph node mapping to test whether spread of the cancer has occurred, with a much lower risk of discomfort and swelling. In addition, major surgical advances include new breast reconstruction techniques such as the skin sparing mastectomy, which have significantly improved the appearance of the breast after mastectomy. There was a time when women were afraid of having breast reconstruction for fear that breast implants could be harmful by causing autoimmune diseases. Many studies of this question now show no harm from implants. Today, the vast majority of women who have had a mastectomy can have some form of breast reconstruction, either with implants or various procedures that use tissue from another area of the body to reconstruct the breast. These approaches have been a significant advance for women who need mastectomy. However, most women today will not require a mastectomy because breast cancer is now found earlier, permitting breast conservation with lumpectomy and radiation. The wide availability of expert radiation centers has given many women the opportunity of replacing mastectomy with breast radiation.

In the past decade, major advances have occurred in the use of chemotherapy and hormonal therapy in treatment of both newly diagnosed breast cancer and recurrent or advanced breast cancer. This has resulted in both improved cure rates and also improved quality of life for breast cancer patients. An important new class of chemotherapy drugs, the taxanes, was developed and is now in widespread use with significant improvement in cure rates and survival. New forms of drugs that exploit biochemical pathways are showing promise to enhance cure and prolong survival with minimal toxicity.

There have also been important changes in the way chemotherapy is now given. Twenty-five years ago, some women received prolonged courses of chemotherapy to prevent relapse. Over time, many clinical trials showed equal effectiveness with much shorter courses of treatment. This shortening of chemotherapy treatment has resulted in less toxicity without lowering cure rates. This process of performing comparitive clinical trials on breast cancer chemotherapy was also very influential in establishing the type of scientific study needed to prove that a cancer treatment was unquestionably effective, rather than relying on intuition or individual experience. Clinical trials in breast cancer have established a firm scientific base that demonstrates that chemotherapy and hormonal therapy improve cure rates.

For women with advanced breast cancer, there have also been major improvements in treatment, leading to improved durations of survival and better quality of life. Newer hormonal therapies have been developed, giving patients more and better options for hormonal treatment. These newer therapies can control breast cancer for longer periods of time and with fewer side effects. Likewise, new chemotherapy drugs such as taxanes, gemcitabine, and capecitabine are effective additions to the chemotherapy armamentarium with high rates of response and very tolerable side effects. The introduction of Herceptin, a new biological agent, has improved survival when combined with chemotherapy in certain groups of patients with advanced breast cancer. A new class of drugs, bisphosphonates, has been introduced to lessen the extent of breast cancer spread into the bones and significantly reduces discomfort as well. The next several years will see the introduction of new and important therapies that are currently making their way down the research pipeline.

Chemotherapy is also now much easier to receive. The immediate toxicities of treatment have been reduced and many of the side effects typically associated with treatment have been ameliorated. This has coincided with the introduction of new medications that prevent nausea and that reduce blood count problems. In the past, these were both major side effects for patients receiving chemotherapy. Solutions for these problems have made chemotherapy easier to take, permitting more patients to receive treatment with a corresponding improvement in survival for all stages of breast cancer.

Newer testing methods on a patient's breast cancer allow doctors to more accurately select treatments for each individual patient. Assays are now routinely used to detect the presence of hormone receptors for estrogen and progesterone on every breast cancer, indicating whether or not a patient is likely to benefit from hormonal treatment. An even more recent test analysis for Her2 identifies which patients are appropriate candidates to receive a new treatment, trastusamab (Herceptin). The recent introduction of molecular analyses is now providing more refined methods for analyzing each individual breast cancer to assess risk and permit more accurate treatment planning. I anticipate that within a few years, these tests and other tests for gene expression will be widely used.

Supportive care is now recognized as having important value in minimizing the distress that goes with the diagnosis of breast cancer. Group and individual session therapy have become widely encouraged and accepted. Such care can help patients through their treatments and have very positive effects on their interactions with family and friends.

There is a bright future for breast cancer care, building on these and other findings discussed in this book. The strategies developed over the last forty years are now bearing fruit, resulting in women being diagnosed with smaller breast cancers, in surgeries that are less disfiguring, and in treatments that are easier to receive, which all lead to higher cure rates. I see new strategies evolving, including targeted therapies in which specific growth pathways within a cancer are blocked; newer hormonal treatments that will prevent breast cancer from growing; a rise in biological methods of cancer treatment; new applications of breast radiation with shorter treatments; new diagnostic tests using information from the human genome project; refinements in breast imaging that more specifically identify whether or not a cancer is present; and new laboratory tests which will distinguish low- from high-risk patients, preventing the use of unneeded chemotherapy.

Breast Cancer: Real Questions, Real Answers tells of the progress that has led to the wide-ranging improvements in breast cancer care that have emerged. Among the topics covered are breast cancer risk and strategies of risk reduction, breast imaging and biopsy, breast surgery, use of chemotherapy and hormonal treatments, new molecular technologies to estimate severity of risk with a new breast cancer, breast reconstructive surgery, radiation therapy, and supportive care.

These are only some of the important issues covered in an informative, reader-friendly way within this book. Unlike many of the books written for women or family members concerned about breast cancer, this book takes the approach that questions are the best way to gather information about this disease. The questions posed are those that I hear most often in taking care of patients. The format of this book can provide a framework to be used for understanding the issues involved in breast cancer care and as a basis for talking with your doctor or family members.

The format of *Breast Cancer: Real Questions, Real Answers* is straightforward and you can skip from question to question and read the parts of interest. Topics can be pursued in sequence or you can skip over topics as needed because the book is internally cross-referenced for ease of navigation. Unlike other books, Dr. Chan includes not only his own view on areas of controversy but also the views of other cancer specialists. This is rather unique in a book for the lay reader.

The sections on chemotherapy and hormonal therapy are very detailed, and provide understanding of this complex topic central to breast cancer care. Lifestyle and psychosocial issues are addressed with practical suggestions and without exaggerating or overstating the benefits of lifestyle change, or of vitamin and supplement alternative therapies. This book is written by an experienced physician and the views expressed are those common among breast cancer experts. It will be useful to those concerned about breast cancer, to women who have developed breast cancer, to their families, and, I suspect, to many physicians concerned with the practical aspects of care.

FRANK E. STOCKDALE, MD, PHD
Professor of Biological Sciences
Maureen Lyles D'Ambrogio Professor of Medicine, Emeritus
Founding Director, Combined Modalities
Breast Cancer Program
Stanford University Cancer Center
Stanford, California

1

❋

How Did I Get
Breast Cancer?

Q *Why did I get breast cancer?*

A There is no simple answer to this question. The American Cancer
Society estimates that in the United States, over 275,000 new cases
of breast cancer will be diagnosed each year. Breast cancer is the leading cause of major cancer in women. Current estimates are that if a
woman in the United States lives to be 100 years old, she will have a
one in eight chance of developing breast cancer.

Q *Is my breast cancer caused by something that I have done?*

A I'll review the main risk factors in this section but the basic answer is
that, in all likelihood, your breast cancer is not caused by something
that you have done, or something that you had much control over.

Q *Then what is the main cause of breast cancer?*

A We know that the major risk factor for breast cancer is being a woman
who was raised in a high socioeconomic country. Women raised in
North America or Western Europe have the highest worldwide risk
for getting breast cancer. Women raised in third world countries have
the lowest worldwide risk. This is the major risk factor and it obviously
isn't under your control.

Q *Why do breast cancer rates differ from one country to another country?*

A The differences are actually very dramatic. Many studies of population trends, called epidemiology studies, show that breast cancer is a disease that occurs much more in developed industrialized countries. The very highest rates of breast cancer occur in North America and Western Europe where breast cancer is 5 times as common as in Asia. This is primarily due to dietary and social factors rather than from inherited risks. We know that breast cancer is not primarily genetic or inherited, as a result of studies that evaluate breast cancer risk in women who immigrate. As an example, breast cancer occurs in a much lower rate in Asia than in the United States. However, Asian American women have breast cancer rates similar to those of American women of European descent.

The reasons are complicated but let me give you a brief summary. It's thought that hormonal stimulation by estrogen during puberty and breast development play an important role in increasing breast cancer rate. In North America and Western Europe, as a result of a high calorie diet and excellent nutrition, puberty occurs several years earlier compared to undeveloped countries. Estrogen stimulates breast development and when puberty occurs earlier, estrogen stimulation of breast tissue occurs earlier as well. Pregnancy and breast-feeding interrupt the estrogen stimulation of breast tissue. In North America and Western Europe, young women tend to delay marriage and childbirth to pursue education and professional opportunities, as opposed to third world countries where multiple pregnancies during teenage years are common. In North America and Western Europe, mothers tend not to breast-feed their infants except for a short period of time, compared to third world countries where breast-feeding commonly extends well beyond one year. Dr. Valerie Beral and her team from Oxford, England, have looked at risk factors and breast cancer in combined studies totaling 150,000 women worldwide. She recently reported that prolonged breast-feeding, as occurs in third world countries, markedly reduces women's chances of getting breast cancer by almost half. Prolonged breast-feeding does this by lowering estrogen levels for long periods of time.

Therefore, higher socioeconomic background leading to early and uninterrupted stimulation of developing breast tissue by estrogen in young women is thought to play a major part in the increased numbers of breast cancer in the United States and other industrialized countries. It seems that the biggest part of the estrogen story is probably during puberty and early adult life and leads to higher risks of

Estimated Breast Cancer Cases/Deaths Worldwide

Region	New Cases 2000	Deaths 2000
Eastern Africa	12,615	6,119
Middle Africa	3,902	1,775
Northern Africa	18,724	8,388
Southern Africa	5,537	2,504
Western Africa	17,389	7,830
Caribbean	6,210	2,310
Central America	18,663	5,888
South America	69,924	22,735
Northern America	202,044	51,184
Eastern Asia	142,656	38,826
South-Eastern Asia	55,907	24,961
South Central Asia	129,620	62,212
Western Asia	20,155	8,459
Eastern Europe	110,975	43,058
Northern Europe	54,551	20,992
Southern Europe	65,284	25,205
Western Europe	115,308	40,443
Australia	12,748	3,427
New Zealand	470	209
Melanesia	62	28
Micronesia	127	58

breast cancer in the later decades, which is when breast cancer usually occurs.

Q *Why do the effects of prolonged and uninterrupted estrogen exposure occur so many years later?*

A Cancers occur as a result of changes in DNA. In essence, DNA is the blueprint plans of your body that controls the growth and function of normal cells. Any error in the DNA, no matter how small, can create a major problem over time. These changes in DNA have been actively studied and are thought to involve multiple cumulative errors, not just one big event. This is why though smoking causes lung cancer, smokers actually don't get lung cancer immediately and the 10 percent of smokers that get lung cancer do so only after many years of smoking. Similarly most women in the United States, although living in a country with higher breast cancer risk, will not actually get breast cancer despite being exposed to the dietary and social risk factors mentioned above. Even though all women growing up in industrialized countries are at higher risk, the reasons why some women get breast cancer while others do not indicate that there are other risk factors that also play a part in breast cancer development.

KEIKO IS FORTY-TWO and Japanese American. She was born in Japan but came to the United States when she was three. She quickly assimilated life in San Francisco and grew up with multicultural friends. Her favorite foods were pizza, hamburgers, fries, and milkshakes. She was a hardworking, diligent student and graduated at the top of her class from U.C. Berkeley. She followed this with an MBA at the University of Southern California.

Hired right out of college by a large regional bank, Keiko worked her way up to an associate vice president position. She married Kevin, a financial analyst for a brokerage firm, when she was thirty-six. They have no children, travel frequently, and are avid supporters of the L.A. Symphony.

Keiko appears composed but with a trace of nervousness. After some casual conversation, I begin to review with her the biopsy results showing an invasive cancer. She interrupts me and ruefully comments, "I just can't believe I have breast cancer. This is totally unbelievable. I feel like I'm in a bad dream and I can't wait to wake up. I try to eat right, don't drink, never smoked. No one in my family has had breast cancer. Actually, I thought Asians usually don't get breast cancer. We have small breasts to begin with. What did I do to cause this?"

During the course of our consultation, I explain to Keiko that she has common misconceptions regarding breast cancer risk. Her main risk factor for getting breast cancer is growing up in a high socioeconomic country,

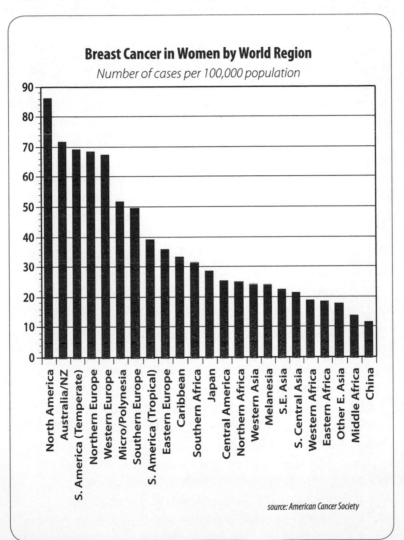

Breast Cancer in Women by World Region

Number of cases per 100,000 population

source: American Cancer Society

not family history, not race, and not breast size. Keiko's socioeconomic background affected the amount of estrogen stimulation she received during puberty and breast development, which is a key factor for breast cancer risk as an adult. Keiko didn't do anything to cause her cancer.

Q *I always thought that breast cancer is inherited and that because no one in my family has had breast cancer that I would not get it. Why is that not true?*

A Contrary to popular belief, most breast cancer is not inherited. Eighty to eighty-five percent of newly diagnosed breast cancer patients do not have a direct relative who has had the disease. About 10 percent of breast cancer is primarily inherited. Two main genes involved in inherited breast cancer have been identified: BRCA1 and BRCA2. BRCA stands for breast cancer susceptibility gene. BRCA will be discussed in more detail in chapter 3.

For most women with breast cancer, no clear hereditary risk can be identified. This is why breast cancer screening is recommended for all women, regardless of family history. All women need mammograms at the appropriate age, not just women who have a family member with breast cancer. The absence of relatives with breast cancer is in no way protective. This is a common misconception.

Q *Now that I have breast cancer, does that mean that my daughter will get it?*

A Probably not. Unless you are in the 10 percent of breast cancers that are clearly familial and usually related to the BRCA genes, your daughter's risk is only slightly elevated compared to the average woman. However, you should still remind your daughter to undergo breast screening and she should discuss the timing of when mammograms should start with her physician.

Q *Was my breast cancer caused by taking estrogen?*

A As mentioned previously, estrogen is certainly important as a risk factor. However the most significant time of risk development probably occurs during breast growth during puberty and young adulthood.

Taking estrogen after menopause has also been identified as a risk factor but a relatively small one in comparison. For example, breast cancer is 5 times more common in the United States than in Thailand, an increase in risk of 500 percent. The magnitude of this difference is much greater than the single digit percentage point difference in breast cancer risk between women who take postmenopausal hormones and women who don't. Taking postmenopausal estrogen is only a very minor risk factor for breast cancer development.

Two studies help to illustrate this point. The first study is called the Nurses' Health Study, which is a long-term study of nurses by Harvard researchers evaluating a number of different women's health issues. The nurses complete regular health questionnaires and their health is monitored over many years. One topic of that study is the relationship between estrogen use after menopause and the development of breast cancer. Nurses were questioned about their use of estrogen and then monitored to see if they developed breast cancer. Nurses who took estrogen after menopause had a risk of breast cancer of about 14 percent. Nurses who never took estrogen after menopause had a risk of breast cancer of about 12 percent. Therefore, although postmenopausal estrogen did increase the risk, the overall increase was relatively small and certainly could not be blamed for the large majority of breast cancers.

A second study that sheds light on the small but consistently established increased risk of breast cancer resulting from postmenopausal estrogen replacement therapy is the current Women's Health Initiative, which is a national study of various health issues in American women. Initial results were reported in 2003. This study also showed that taking estrogen after menopause increased the risk of breast cancer. However the risk was relatively small, estimated at about 0.1 percent (one tenth of one percent) per year of estrogen use.

It's important for patients who have taken estrogen to know that there is a risk associated with postmenopausal estrogen. However, it's also important to keep in mind that the documented increase in risk is quite small, and therefore not likely to be the cause of their breast cancer. The much more substantial estrogen risk occurred decades earlier and was the uninterrupted estrogen stimulation during puberty, breast development, and young adulthood as a result of diet and social factors related to growing up in the United States. This is not something that any woman with breast cancer could have consciously controlled. I know that many of my patients who have taken hormone replacement therapy after menopause blame themselves for their breast cancer. This is an incorrect view and I hope that you can now see that the cause of your breast cancer was really beyond your control.

Q *Several months before I was diagnosed, I fell and injured my breast. The cancer is right where it hurt. Could this injury have contributed to my getting breast cancer?*

A No. There is no scientific data to support injury or trauma as a risk factor. The development of breast cancer from the first cancer cell to diagnosis usually takes years, and therefore events occurring within the recent months or the past year are not important, because the cancer was already present.

For example, the growth of a breast cancer to 1 cm (centimeter) in size, a diameter about the width of the fingernail on your little finger, involves the growth of about one billion cancer cells. Given what is known about breast cancer cell growth rates, the time it takes to grow from a single cell to one billion cells would be on average about six to eight years. Of course in rare instances, there are breast cancers that are very aggressive and can grow much more quickly.

Q *I hate my job and this past year my husband and I have been having some problems. Is my breast cancer caused by stress?*

A There are no accepted scientific studies demonstrating that stress causes cancer. Much has been written about stress and the immune system, but breast cancer isn't thought to arise primarily from a breakdown in the immune system. Because your breast cancer comes from your own breast tissue, your cancer has all the same immune signals of your normal breast cells (with very minor exceptions). Therefore, the problem is that your immune system isn't able to identify that the breast cancer cell shouldn't be there and doesn't eliminate it. The overall functional status of your immune system is fine. Again, it's important to recognize that breast cancer takes years to grow to a size that can be detected, so a recent stressful time or a recent traumatic event would have occurred after the cancer had already been present and growing for some time.

ROBIN IS IN her late sixties and visibly upset. Nine months ago, she found a lump in her breast that didn't seem to change over time. She thought it was a cyst. Unfortunately, it was a 1 cm breast cancer and she's scheduled to have a lumpectomy and sentinel node biopsy.

When I ask her how she's doing, she tearfully exclaims, "I just knew something like this was going to happen. I feel like my life's a wreck and I've never been under such stress. In July, my husband's work told him that he'd probably lose his job unless he takes early retirement. My boss has been out half the year because of a car accident so I'm trying to do my work and his. On top of that, my daughter's husband recently left her and the kids. This entire year has been simply terrible. I knew the stress was going to cause something like this."

I sympathize with Robin's problems at home and at work, but I also explain to her that stress didn't cause her cancer. Breast cancer generally grows fairly slowly. Her cancer was growing microscopically and undetectably for more than five years, and clearly started growing prior to this very difficult time in her life.

It's important for Robin to understand that the unfortunate personal events that are occurring at this time in her life aren't causing her cancer or else she will be needlessly paralyzed with fear that daily-life stress will make her cancer situation worse and increase her chances of relapse. During our visit, I try to ensure that she understands that stress doesn't cause cancer or cancer relapse. Given the relatively small size of her cancer, I feel confident that Robin has a good chance for complete recovery. I convey my optimism to her and she starts to feel more hopeful.

Q *I have breast implants. Did they cause my breast cancer?*
A A number of studies have looked at this issue and the answer is that breast implants don't cause breast cancer. Breast implants can make

it harder to find the cancer using mammogram because the implants shield some areas of the breast from being well seen. This is relevant because so many women have breast implants. In 2002, there were over 250,000 breast augmentations in the United States.

Implants and breast cancer were the subject of a recent study by Professor Diana Migliorette from the University of Washington, Seattle. She and her team found that even though mammograms were somewhat less able to diagnose breast cancer in women with implants, this didn't affect the stage of the cancer, and the breast cancer in patients with implants was not more severe at the time of diagnosis compared to women without implants. This may be because women with implants tend to have less breast tissue and the implant provides a firm platform so that self-detection of breast cancer is easier.

Q *I take one or two drinks on occasion. What is the relationship between alcohol and breast cancer?*

A There is a small effect between daily alcohol intake and getting breast cancer. Whether or not drinking contributes to breast cancer directly or whether drinking is related to other important lifestyle factors is not clear. This was analyzed by Dr. Smith-Warner, an epidemiologist, and her team at Harvard who reviewed a number of pooled studies on alcohol and breast cancer. They reported that with increasing daily alcohol intake, there was a corresponding increase in risk of getting breast cancer. The type of alcohol didn't seem to make a difference.

Alcohol and breast cancer risk was also a part of Dr. Beral's Oxford study. That study also showed that although alcohol was a risk factor, overall its impact is relatively small. She reported that if alcohol were completely eliminated, the incidence of breast cancer would drop by only 4 percent. It's possible that the increased breast cancer risk is related to higher estrogen levels in postmenopausal patients who drink alcohol daily. Women who drink infrequently were considered non-drinkers and it's unlikely that occasional alcohol intake increases breast cancer risk in a meaningful way.

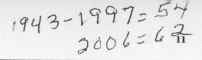

11

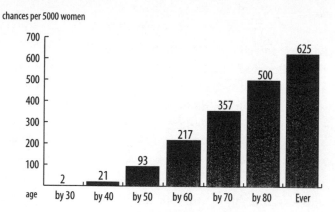

A Woman's Chances of Breast Cancer Increase with Age

chances per 5000 women

age	by 30	by 40	by 50	by 60	by 70	by 80	Ever
	2	21	93	217	357	500	625

Cumulative risk of breast cancer increases with age.
Most breast cancers occur after age 50.

from Feuer EJ et al: Probability of Developing or Dying of Cancer. Version 4.0 Bethesda MD. National Cancer Institute. 1999

Q *Are diet, obesity, and lack of exercise risk factors?*

A Yes, they are considered minor risk factors. They are interrelated and seem to increase breast cancer risk by causing higher estrogen levels that stimulate growth of breast tissue. Many studies show that being overweight, eating a high-fat diet, and having a sedentary lifestyle slightly increase breast cancer risk. On these lifestyle issues, it's important not to get carried away, and keep in mind that the demonstrated increases in risk are very small. It appears that obesity tends to slightly increase circulating estrogen levels. Body fat contains an enzyme called aromatase, which can make estrogen, and in postmenopausal patients, this can cause slightly higher estrogen levels. The amount of increase in estrogen is much lower than the amount contained in estrogen replacement therapy for menopause, and I have already discussed how relatively small a contribution that makes to the overall development of breast cancer. These are minor risk factors rather than major ones. The lifestyle factors of diet in later adult life, obesity, and exercise only alter an individual's breast cancer risk by very small degrees.

Q *Should I have eaten better? Should I have exercised more?*

A Again, the time that your diet was probably most important was during puberty and teenage years, decades before your getting breast cancer. A high-fat, high-calorie diet when growing up can result in an earlier puberty with earlier onset of breast development. This is the main reason that dietary studies in different countries demonstrate different rates of breast cancer.

Recent diet during the ten years preceding the diagnosis of breast cancer probably is unimportant for the following reasons. It is similar to the case of smoking and lung cancer; it takes many years of cigarette exposure before the development of lung cancer. Lung cancer doesn't occur after smoking for five years but after smoking for decades. In breast cancer, diet for the several years prior to diagnosis is not relevant because the cancer has usually been present for a number of years before growing large enough to become detectable. Studies do show that diets having higher fat content during premenopausal years do lead to a higher chance of breast cancer in the postmenopausal years.

However, attempts to lower breast cancer risk by lowering dietary fat without corresponding weight loss have not lowered the rates of breast cancer. This has been very frustrating to experts who perform these studies. Some experts feel that the problem with these studies was that the fat content was not lowered enough. What is more likely is that diet later in life, during postmenopausal years, probably has a minor impact compared to the more major risk factors we've already discussed.

There are studies indicating that being overweight and not exercising may slightly increase breast cancer risk. This seems to be because obesity and a sedentary lifestyle are associated with higher postmenopausal estrogen levels. Again, I must emphasize that although these factors have been extensively studied and reported on, the overall effects are quite small. The effects of adult lifestyle on breast cancer risk are relatively minor compared to the major risk factor of being a woman raised in North America or Western Europe. The effects of diet and lifestyle during adolescence and young adulthood are huge compared to the small differences made by diet, obesity, and sedentary lifestyle decades later.

Q *So it seems that my family genes and my current lifestyle are probably not to be blamed for my breast cancer?*

A That's correct. It's very unlikely that your breast cancer results from something that you have done or that you could have controlled. All the risk factors you could have controlled as an adult play a relatively small role in your having gotten breast cancer. In addition to all the turmoil that your illness is causing you, you should not feel at all guilty that this is something that you have brought on yourself. Now, let's concentrate our energies on getting you well.

2

※

What Is Breast Cancer?

Q *What is breast cancer?*

A Breast cancer is a growth of abnormal tissue within the breast that is dangerous because it causes damage by invading and disrupting normal breast tissue. Even more significant is its tendency to spread and damage other organs. Breast cancer develops from normal breast tissue, from the structures within the breast that are responsible for making breast milk (the lobules) or carrying the breast milk to the nipple (the ducts). There are two important characteristics of any cancer that make it very different from normal tissue. The first is that cancer cells don't stop growing and essentially have no "off switch," a process which scientists call apoptosis. Normal cells do stop growing when growth is supposed to be completed, such as cells of the skin that mend to cover a cut. The second important characteristic of cancer is that cancer cells also have ability to spread to other areas of the body via the blood and lymph systems, a process called metastasis. It is these two characteristics of cancer, immortality and the tendency to spread, which make cancer dangerous.

Normal Breast Anatomy

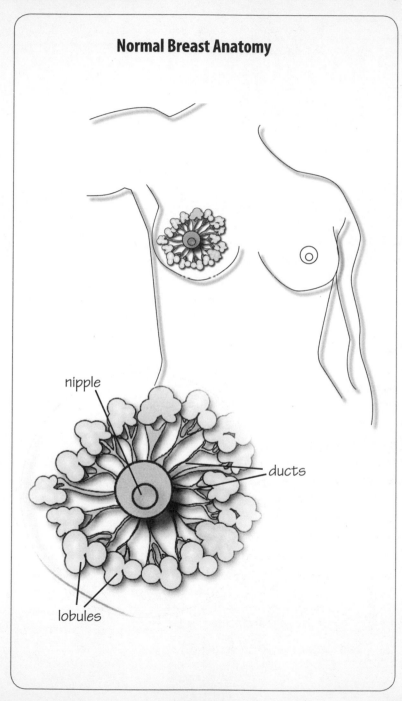

nipple

ducts

lobules

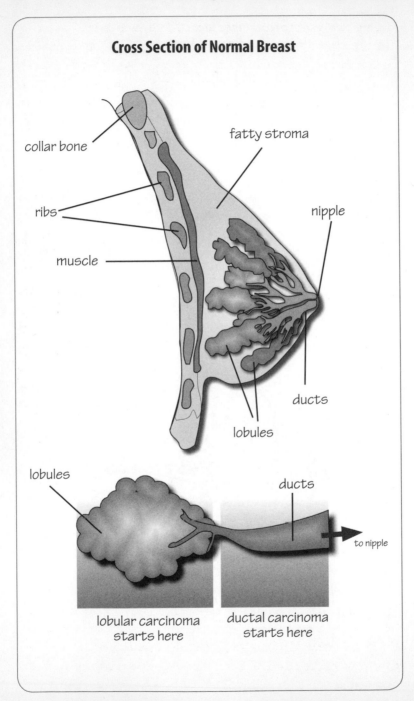

Cross Section of Normal Breast

collar bone

fatty stroma

ribs

nipple

muscle

ducts

lobules

lobules

ducts

to nipple

lobular carcinoma
starts here

ductal carcinoma
starts here

Q *Is every cancer that occurs in the breast, breast cancer?*

A There are rare cancers that start in the breast but are not considered breast cancer. Breast cancer comes from either the breast ducts or the lobules. If a cancer starts from an immune cell called a lymphocyte, the cancer is called a lymphoma. If a cancer starts from muscle components that line blood vessels or structural supporting cells or fat, the cancer is called a sarcoma. These cancers rarely start in the breast and are not considered breast cancer because they can start anywhere within the body and aren't specific cancers to the breast. However, breast cancer only starts from the cells that line the ducts (ductal carcinoma) or from the cells that make up the lobules (lobular carcinoma).

Q *What is the most common type of breast cancer?*

A More than 80 percent of breast cancers are ductal carcinomas. The cancer gets its name because it originates in the breast ducts, the tubes that carry milk to the nipple during breast-feeding. The word carcinoma is the technical term for cancer. If the cancer grows through the duct wall into the fatty tissue of the breast, it is called invasive or infiltrating ductal carcinoma. Infiltrating ductal carcinoma is the most common type of invasive breast cancer and is characterized by having ductal cancer cells that have penetrated the duct wall. When penetration or invasion occurs, the cancer becomes more dangerous because it can then spread to other areas of the body.

Q *What is DCIS?*

A DCIS stands for ductal carcinoma in situ. In situ is Latin for " in place." This means that cancer cells are present and growing within the duct, but the cancer cells do not penetrate the duct wall. It is important to know that DCIS is noninvasive so the risk of spread to other areas of the body is extremely low. DCIS is often discovered by mammogram although sometimes it can also be found as a lump. The main problem with DCIS is that if it isn't properly treated, over years it can develop into invasive cancer. Fortunately, the large majority of women with DCIS will never develop invasive breast cancer, and therefore the treatment strategy for DCIS is different from that of invasive ductal carcinoma.

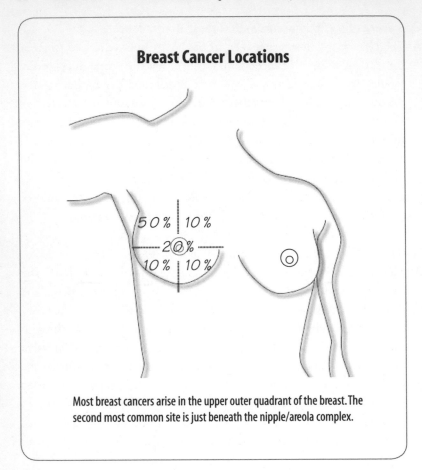

Breast Cancer Locations

50% 10%

20%

10% 10%

Most breast cancers arise in the upper outer quadrant of the breast. The second most common site is just beneath the nipple/areola complex.

Q *What is lobular carcinoma?*

A This is breast cancer that starts in the lobules of the breast, the structures at the end of the ducts. During breast-feeding, breast milk is made from the lobules and flows through the ducts into the nipple. If you can picture the lobules and duct structure of the breast as being similar to a stalk of broccoli, the lobules would be the tufts and the ducts would be the branches.

Lobular carcinoma also occurs in two varieties, an invasive form and an in situ (noninvasive) form. Again, having invasive lobular carcinoma is much more serious than having lobular carcinoma in situ because lobular carcinoma in situ will not spread.

There are differences in behavior between invasive ductal and invasive

Evolution of Ductal Carcinoma

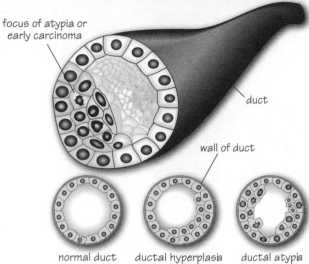

focus of atypia or early carcinoma

duct

wall of duct

normal duct   ductal hyperplasia   ductal atypia

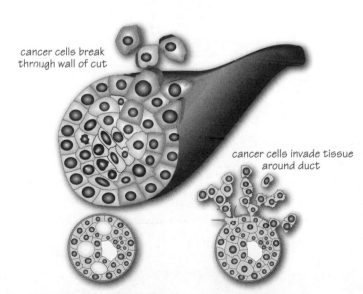

cancer cells break through wall of cut

cancer cells invade tissue around duct

ductal carcinoma in situ (DCIS)   invasive ductal carcinoma

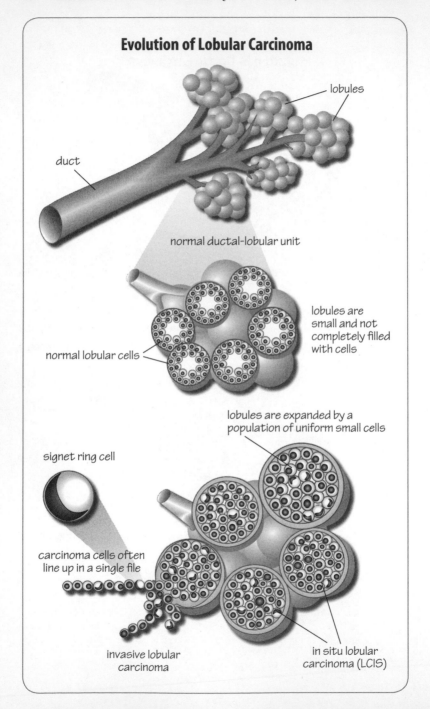

Evolution of Lobular Carcinoma

lobules

duct

normal ductal-lobular unit

lobules are small and not completely filled with cells

normal lobular cells

lobules are expanded by a population of uniform small cells

signet ring cell

carcinoma cells often line up in a single file

invasive lobular carcinoma

in situ lobular carcinoma (LCIS)

lobular carcinoma. Invasive lobular carcinoma has a higher chance of being bilateral, occurring in both breasts, compared to invasive ductal cancers. Lobular cancers are also harder to see on mammogram and are the most commonly missed breast cancer on mammogram. This is because of how lobular cancers grow, in thin tentacles between normal breast structures, causing less breast reaction. When an invasive lobular carcinoma is visible on mammogram, often the size will be underestimated. Studies are currently in progress to see if the size of lobular cancers is more accurately measured by MRI scanning.

Q *What is LCIS?*

A LCIS stands for lobular carcinoma in situ. The cancer cells are present and growing within the lobules, the milk producing structures (the tufts at the ends of the broccoli stalk), but have not yet penetrated through the lobule wall into the breast fat. LCIS is not treated like breast cancer. It is thought to represent a marker for having a higher chance of developing breast cancer. When LCIS is diagnosed, it's estimated that the chance of getting an invasive breast cancer is about 1 percent per year. It's important to note that if an invasive cancer starts, it can occur in either breast, not just the breast with LCIS. Because of this, some women elect to have bilateral mastectomies, removal of the breasts, but most women choose to continue breast cancer screening with yearly mammograms. It is not thought that the LCIS itself turns into breast cancer, because most breast cancers occurring in relationship to LCIS are ductal and not lobular. Therefore it is considered a risk factor for invasive breast cancer but it is not essential to remove all the LCIS from the breast. Often when LCIS is present, it is scattered throughout the breast rather than being localized to an area easily removed without mastectomy.

When LCIS is found on a biopsy, it's usually because of an abnormality found on a mammogram. It's reasonable to remove the mammogram abnormality to make sure that there isn't a more significant cancer problem present such as DCIS or even invasive cancer. Up to 15 percent of the time, when a needle biopsy shows LCIS, and the mammogram abnormality is excised, a more serious breast cancer is found.

AMELIA HAS NEW calcifications on her mammogram. Her mother is a breast cancer survivor and Amelia is very diligent about breast screening. No breast mass can be felt and her ultrasound is normal. A stereotactic biopsy is performed which shows LCIS, lobular carcinoma in situ.

It's our first visit, and I explain to Amelia the meaning of her biopsy, which shows a noninvasive cancer. The cancer cells are contained within the lobules, which are the milk glands of her breast. I draw a diagram to help her better understand and explain that having LCIS isn't immediately dangerous. However, the affected area requires excision by a surgeon because infrequently, a more serious condition is hidden within the LCIS.

Fortunately, as is usually the case, Amelia's surgical excision reveals only LCIS, and the margins are involved with LCIS. In our post-surgery visit, I inform her that although some LCIS remains in her breast, it doesn't require further surgery for removal. Having LCIS increases her risk of breast cancer and the cancer can develop in either breast. Taking Tamoxifen can reduce that risk by almost half. She agrees to take it and she'll also continue monthly self-exam and yearly mammograms.

Over a twenty-year span, by taking Tamoxifen for five years, Amelia's chance of getting invasive breast cancer by the age of eighty-three are lowered from 20 percent to 10 percent. The odds are very good that she won't get an invasive breast cancer in her lifetime.

Q *What is tubular carcinoma?*

A This is a breast cancer that originates from the ducts. Under the microscope, a tubular cancer appears almost like normal breast ducts and pathologists sometimes have difficulty in determining if a cancer is present. Tubular carcinoma tends to grow slowly and to spread infrequently. It is one of the slowest-growing breast cancers. This type of cancer is not common, occurring about 1 percent of the time.

Q *What is a medullary carcinoma?*

A This cancer makes up about 5 percent of breast cancers. It typically has a faster growth rate and often is discovered as a lump in the breast. Most medullary carcinomas are negative for estrogen and progesterone receptors. This can be important and I discuss the significance of this point in chapter 6.

Q *What is a mucinous carcinoma?*
A This type of cancer occurs infrequently, about 2 percent of the time. Mucinous carcinoma tends to grow slowly and therefore is considered a more favorable type of breast cancer.

Q *What is ADH?*
A ADH stands for atypical ductal hyperplasia and isn't a cancer. In ADH, there are abnormal cells in the ducts, but the cells are not quite abnormal enough for the pathologist to diagnose DCIS. Like DCIS, ADH leads to an increased chance of getting breast cancer. Usually ADH occurs throughout the breast so that, unlike typical DCIS, there is not one specific area that can be removed. According to Dr. David Page at Vanderbilt University, ADH can lead to a risk of breast cancer at a rate of less than 1 percent per year. If ADH is diagnosed by needle biopsy, the mammogram abnormality should be excised to make sure that there isn't a cancer there. When an area of DCIS is found on mammogram and subsequently removed by lumpectomy, about 15 percent of the time either DCIS or an invasive cancer will also be found. ADH is part of a continuum in the development of invasive breast cancer. The sequence of developing a breast cancer is normal cells change to ADH, which then change to DCIS, and then lastly become an infiltrating ductal carcinoma. This sequence takes many years to develop.

MARGARITA IS FIFTY-FIVE and in great health. She's been on estrogen replacement for the last three years. Her current mammogram has an area of change, new calcifications, in her left breast compared to last year. Core needle biopsies are performed.

Margarita's biopsies contain three different abnormalities; intermediate grade DCIS, a small area of microinvasion, and ADH. A biopsy having more than one abnormality can confuse patients. Margarita's biopsy results are not immediately dangerous but in time could lead to an invasive cancer if not properly treated.

It's not uncommon to have mixed abnormalities on a breast biopsy or within a lumpectomy specimen. Within any cancer, there are different areas that change at different rates over many months, some becoming more abnormal and potentially more dangerous.

I ask Margarita to stop taking estrogen and I recommend that she undergo a lumpectomy. I also let her know that sometimes, infrequently, the lumpectomy specimen will reveal a more serious condition such as an invasive cancer. I also encourage her not to worry because she has an excellent chance of being well.

Q *What is Paget's disease?*

A This is the development of breast cancer cells within the ducts within the nipple. The cancer is generally in situ, noninvasive. When Paget's disease occurs, it's important to make sure that there isn't an underlying invasive cancer deeper within the breast, which sometimes occurs. An underlying invasive cancer can push cancer cells up the ductal system into the nipple resulting in Paget's disease. Paget's disease of the nipple is often discovered when a woman finds crusting of the nipple, sometimes with discomfort or itching, sometimes with a discolored discharge from the nipple.

Q *What is inflammatory breast cancer?*

A Inflammatory breast cancer is a particularly aggressive form of breast cancer that results when breast cancer cells are spreading through the lymph system of the breast in amounts large enough to cause lymph blockage. As a result, the cancer cells back up toward the skin and cause redness and swelling of the skin of the breast. The skin has a quality like an orange peel and there's a term used to describe the skin texture, *peau d'orange*, which means orange peel in French. The significance of inflammatory breast cancer is that it's a very aggressive form of invasive breast cancer. Chemotherapy is almost always used first, to reduce the size of the cancer before the patient undergoes surgery, which is usually a mastectomy. I discuss the importance of sequencing treatments in chapter 14.

3

·※·

Is Breast Cancer Inherited?

Q *I thought that if no relative in my family had breast cancer, I wouldn't need to worry about it.*

A That's a common belief and it's untrue. As previously mentioned, 80 to 85 percent of new patients with breast cancer don't have a family member with breast cancer. Inherited breast cancer makes up only about 10 percent of all new breast cancer patients. As I discussed in chapter 1, the main risk factor for getting breast cancer is being a woman who grew up in a high socioeconomic part of the world such as North America or Western Europe.

Q *So hereditary factors aren't important?*

A Hereditary factors can be important. For about 80 to 85 percent of new breast cancer patients, they just aren't the most important factor. There exists well-documented breast and ovarian cancer families. The increased cancers are caused by an abnormal gene that controls growth patterns of breast and ovary tissue. The abnormality within the gene is called a mutation.

The mutated gene has a dominant transmission pattern. That means that having only one copy of the abnormal gene from either parent can put a woman at risk. A parent carrying this gene has a 50 percent chance of passing it to an offspring. A mother can pass it to her son, who can then pass it on to his daughter. In some of these families, there are family members with breast and/or ovarian cancer within every generation.

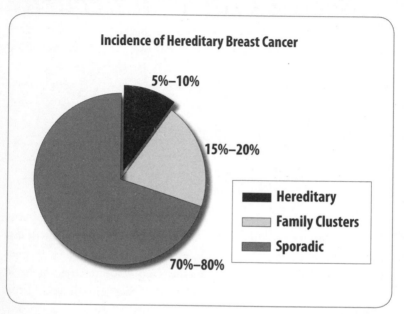

Incidence of Hereditary Breast Cancer

5%–10%

15%–20%

70%–80%

Hereditary
Family Clusters
Sporadic

Q *Can this gene be tested for?*

A Yes, there is a test for it, but it's important to keep in mind that the test is only meaningful if the results are abnormal, because not all the genes causing hereditary breast cancer have been discovered. The genes that currently have an existing test are BRCA1 and BRCA2. BRCA stands for breast cancer susceptibility gene. The numbers 1 and 2 indicate that two genes have been identified. The test is done through a blood test and unfortunately is expensive, around $3,000.

Q *Does insurance pay for this test?*

A Most insurance plans will pay for it if there is a significant family history. If you are considering the test, you should have it pre-authorized by your insurance company. In general, to undergo BRCA testing, you should have had at least one other relative with either breast or ovarian cancer. Otherwise your chances of carrying an abnormal BRCA1 or BRCA2 gene are low.

CANDACE IS FORTY-FIVE, the mother of three, and a college counselor. Her husband, Brad, and her sister from New York accompany her to my office. Candace has a 1.4 cm invasive ductal cancer diagnosed by mammogram.

"Does anyone in your family have breast or ovarian cancer?" Candace replies, "No, not really, no one that I can think of." As I begin another question, her sister interrupts, "What about Aunt Sadie?" Candace answers, "That doesn't count, she's on Dad's side of the family. No one's had breast cancer on Mom's side."

It turns out that Aunt Sadie is now sixty-four and had breast cancer when she was forty. In addition, her daughter was recently diagnosed with ovarian cancer at the age of forty-three. The family is Jewish and from Western Europe.

I review with them that inherited breast and ovarian cancer syndromes can be passed down from either the mother or father. I suggest that as part of her initial evaluation, we include a blood test for BRCA testing. Test results can take four to five weeks. It's important for Candace and her sister to know how having a BRCA mutation might affect her treatment options and what other implications it might have regarding her health as well as her sister's. Genetic counseling is helpful. I recommend to Candace that she proceed with a lumpectomy and sentinel node biopsy now, and that we re-evaluate the situation if the BRCA test comes back abnormal. If Candace is BRCA positive, she would be considered for more intensive screening or preventative surgeries.

Q *If I have breast cancer and also have just one other relative with breast or ovarian cancer, what are my chances of having an abnormal gene in a test?*

A This actually has been studied and the chances are relatively low. Dr. Kathleen Malone and her team at the University of Washington, Seattle, looked at women under the age of thirty-five with newly diagnosed breast cancer. Their rate of BRCA abnormality was only 6.2 percent. They also looked at newly diagnosed breast cancer in women under the age of forty-five who had one other relative who also had had breast cancer. In that group the rate of BRCA abnormality was 7.2 percent.

A similar analysis was performed by Dr. Julian Peto and her team from the Institute of Cancer Research in England. They found that women diagnosed with breast cancer before the age of thirty-six had a 5.9 percent chance of a BRCA abnormality. These percentages are actually lower than expected because hereditary breast cancers do tend to occur at a younger age. Study results like this suggest the likelihood that there are other genes of importance that are yet to be found. Researchers at UCLA have found that if a newly diagnosed breast cancer patient has a relative who developed breast cancer at a young age, that the chance of BRCA abnormality is somewhat higher and may approach 20 percent.

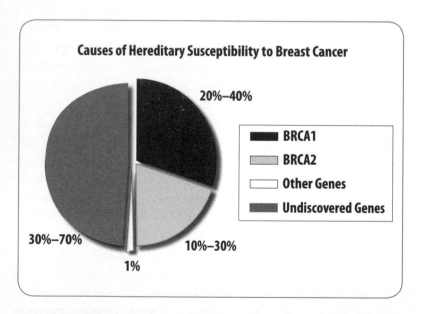

Causes of Hereditary Susceptibility to Breast Cancer

20%–40%

- ■ BRCA1
- ▨ BRCA2
- ☐ Other Genes
- ■ Undiscovered Genes

30%–70%

10%–30%

1%

Q *Why should I consider having BRCA testing?*
A Some mutations of BRCA have high lifetime risks of breast and ovarian cancer. Fortunately, these mutations represent the minority

of known BRCA mutations. Several hundred mutations have been discovered and many of these mutations have no known risk associated with them. They are considered minor mutations that don't affect the function of the gene and therefore probably don't increase breast cancer risk. However there are some mutations that are known to be high risk, with lifetime risks of breast cancer approaching 80 percent and ovarian cancer approaching 40 percent.

A genetic counselor can be helpful in both discussing whether testing should be done and also in explaining the results of the test. This type of service is usually offered at major cancer centers and university hospitals.

Women who carry these mutations require special monitoring (MRI of the breast and transvaginal ultrasound of the ovaries) and some women choose to have preventative surgeries. These surgeries can include removal of normal breasts (prophylactic mastectomies) and preventative removal of normal ovaries using a small incision and a scope (laparoscopic oophorectomy).

Q *For BRCA carriers, are these preventative surgeries effective?*

A Yes, preventative surgeries are very effective in markedly reducing risk. Studies of women carrying BRCA mutations show that preventative mastectomies reduce a woman's risk of breast cancer by over 90 percent and that removal of the ovaries significantly reduces the risk of both breast cancer and ovarian cancer. However, despite the preventative surgeries, the risk of breast and ovarian cancer is never completely eliminated, because even after surgery, there remain small amounts of tissue at risk under the mastectomy scar and within the abdomen.

After a mastectomy, there's still a tiny amount of breast tissue left behind under the skin flaps that make up the surgical scar. Monitoring the mastectomy scar is important because a breast cancer can still occur in this area. Similarly, after preventative removal of the ovaries, there are also small amounts of tissue at risk remaining within the abdominal cavity. This is because the tissue that covers the surface of the ovaries also lines the abdominal cavity. This tissue, called epithelium, can infrequently turn into a cancer that behaves

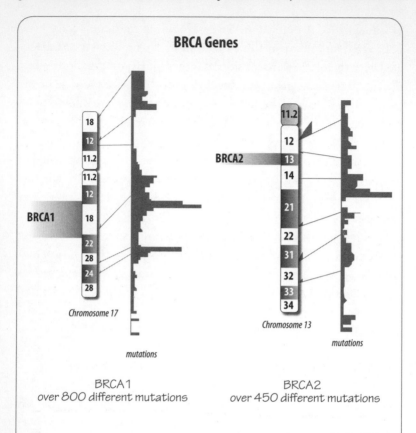

BRCA Genes

BRCA1
Chromosome 17

mutations

BRCA2
Chromosome 13

mutations

BRCA1
over 800 different mutations

BRCA2
over 450 different mutations

Understanding the functions of the proteins made by the BRCA1 and BRCA2 genes has helped scientists understand how mutations in these genes increase the risk of breast and ovarian cancer.

BRCA1 and BRCA2 genes are called "tumor suppressor genes" because they suppress the development of cancer. The proteins encoded by BRCA1 and BRCA2 genes prevent cells from becoming malignant by helping to repair mutations that occur in other genes.

Ordinarily, there is only a one-in-a-million chance that a specific tumor suppressor gene will mutate in a cell. Even if this happens, the tumor suppressing function of the gene is maintained because each cell has a backup copy of the gene on a second duplicate chromosome. The function of the gene is completely lost only if the backup copy is also lost in the same cell.

The majority of the mutations are unique, so that each affected family tends to have its own "private" mutation. A few mutations have been identified in specific populations, such as individuals of Ashkenazi Jewish descent.

Prevalence of Deleterious Mutations in BRCA1 and BRCA2 by Personal and Family History of Cancer in Women

Patient History	Family History (Includes at least one first or second degree relative)					
	No breast CA <50; no ovarian CA in any relative	Breast Cancer <50 in one relative; no ovarian cancer in any relative	Breast Cancer <50 in more than one relative; no ovarian cancer in any relative	Ovarian cancer at any age in one relative; no breast cancer <50 in any relative	Ovarian cancer in more than one relative; no breast cancer <50 in any relative	Breast cancer <50 and ovarian cancer in any age
No breast cancer or ovarian cancer	3.4%	4.5%	9.1%	5.3%	8.9%	14.0%
Breast cancer before ≥ 50	2.9%	7.5%	11.1%	5.6%	13.3%	18.2%
Breast cancer <50	7.3%	17.4%	32.5%	18.5%	28.2%	42.1%
Ovarian cancer at any age; no breast cancer	9.8%	24.3%	42.2%	21.7%	37.4%	50.0%
Breast Cancer ≥ 50 and ovarian cancer at any age	14.8%	29.2%	42.9%	27.0%	53.8%	63.3%
Breast cancer < 50 and ovarian cancer at any age	53.4%	60.0%	76.9%	66.7%	71.4%	78.8%

Modified from Frank TS, Critchfield GC. Clinical Perinatology 2001; 2:395-406 and Myriad Genetic Laboratories; updated Spring 2004. Table does not include individuals of Ashkenazi ancestry.

Sample Pedigree Map in a Family Affected with BRCA1 Gene Mutation

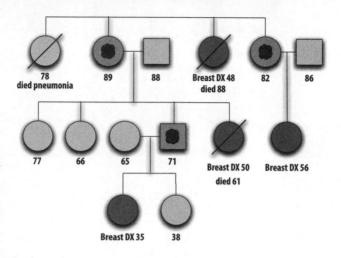

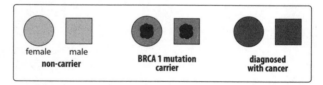

The patient in question is indicated at the bottom left, a woman with breast cancer at the age of 35. The pedigree indicates that she has a strong family history of breast cancer on her father's side including an aunt and grand-aunt and that the gene was passed to her from her father who inherited it from his mother.

biologically like ovarian cancer. So rarely, in the absence of ovaries, an ovarian-type cancer can start within the lining of the abdomen called the peritoneum, and it behaves exactly like ovarian cancer and we treat it with ovarian cancer therapies.

Q *Are there other options besides preventative surgery for BRCA carriers?*

A For breast cancer, an antiestrogen pill called Tamoxifen, which has the brand name Nolvadex, is approved for use to reduce breast cancer risk. It seems to reduce breast cancer in women with BRCA2 mutations, but whether it reduces risk in women with BRCA1 mutations is less clear. A number of studies now suggest that adding breast MRI screening to the mammogram and breast ultrasound is beneficial in women with BRCA mutations. At UCLA the screening procedure for women with BRCA mutations is yearly MRI with mammograms alternating every six months with breast ultrasound. The MRI and mammograms complement each other as different ways to visualize the breast.

Attempts to develop screening tests for ovarian cancer have unfortunately been fairly unsuccessful so far. The two screening tests currently available for ovarian cancer are the transvaginal ultrasound of the ovaries, in which an ultrasound probe is placed into the vagina, and CA-125, a blood test for an ovarian cancer tumor marker. A number of studies have been performed using these tests to screen for ovarian cancer and they have been found to be disappointing. Both tests seem to be unreliable and when ovarian cancer is detected by these screening tests, often it is already advanced. Between the two tests, transvaginal ultrasound is probably the better screening test although both are usually performed in an attempt to screen high-risk ovarian patients.

I generally give my patients who are BRCA carriers the choice of either preventative mastectomies or Tamoxifen with breast screening (including MRI), while simultaneously recommending that the ovaries be preventatively removed by laparoscopy. Removal of the ovaries reduces the risk of breast cancer and eliminates the need to try to screen for ovarian cancer. I only recommend ovarian screening in women who are attempting to have children and want to delay removal of their ovaries. When the family is completed, I then recommend preventative surgery.

KARLA IS THIRTY-TWO and she is BRCA positive. Several years ago, her oldest sister had breast cancer at thirty-nine. Their aunt had breast cancer at sixty-eight. Karla's sister tested positive for BRCA with a major mutation. Unfortunately, Karla has also tested positive for the same BRCA abnormality. Myriad Genetics, the company performing the test, reports that Karla's mutation gives her a 60 to 80 percent lifetime risk of breast cancer and a 20 to 40 percent lifetime risk of ovarian cancer.

Karla is a homemaker, and has a four-year-old daughter. She and her husband, Bill, an aerospace engineer, are seeing me to discuss the BRCA results and her options for treatment. As I give her the genetic test results, she begins to panic. She requests an immediate double mastectomy and removal of her ovaries. I explain to her that that is certainly an option, but her short-term risk of breast cancer is probably no greater than 2 to 3 percent per year. And her chance of getting ovarian cancer is about 2 percent before the age of forty. I present to her a possible alternative option to immediate mastectomies and removal of ovaries.

Karla and Bill really want one more child. I recommend that they attempt to have a child this year. Then, sometime after delivery, Karla will have her ovaries removed because there isn't a reliable screening test for ovarian cancer. The surgery will also help her by lowering her chance of getting breast cancer. Additionally, she would then take Tamoxifen, which might further reduce her breast cancer risk. I would also add MRI breast screening to mammograms and breast ultrasounds for early detection.

Although Karla would be taking a chance regarding breast cancer, we could monitor developments over the next five to seven years regarding breast screening or maybe even BRCA genetic treatments, and delay preventative mastectomies for now.

After some discussion with Bill, Karla makes her decision. "Obviously, I'm scared. But we really want another kid. And I understand that there is some risk. But if you think about it, everything in life has some risk. I think

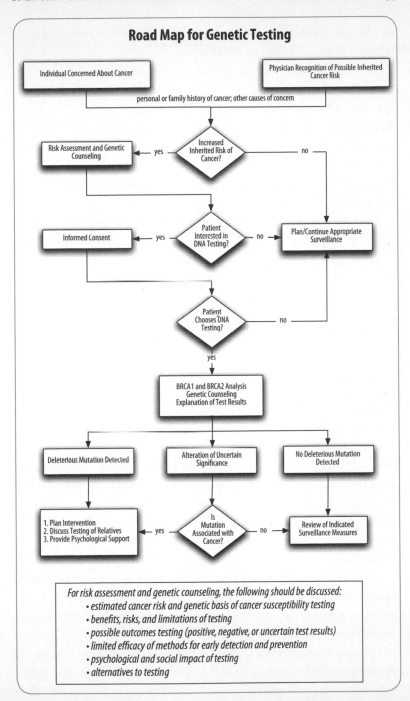

Road Map for Genetic Testing

Individual Concerned About Cancer

Physician Recognition of Possible Inherited Cancer Risk

personal or family history of cancer; other causes of concern

Increased Inherited Risk of Cancer?

Risk Assessment and Genetic Counseling — yes

no

Patient Interested in DNA Testing?

Informed Consent — yes

no → Plan/Continue Appropriate Surveillance

Patient Chooses DNA Testing?

no

yes

BRCA1 and BRCA2 Analysis
Genetic Counseling
Explanation of Test Results

Deleterious Mutation Detected

Alteration of Uncertain Significance

No Deleterious Mutation Detected

1. Plan Intervention
2. Discuss Testing of Relatives
3. Provide Psychological Support

yes — Is Mutation Associated with Cancer? — no → Review of Indicated Surveillance Measures

For risk assessment and genetic counseling, the following should be discussed:
- *estimated cancer risk and genetic basis of cancer susceptibility testing*
- *benefits, risks, and limitations of testing*
- *possible outcomes testing (positive, negative, or uncertain test results)*
- *limited efficacy of methods for early detection and prevention*
- *psychological and social impact of testing*
- *alternatives to testing*

if I can have another kid, and also avoid mastectomies at least for a while, that would be great. Let's go with the plan."

Q *Are there any reasons to not have BRCA testing?*

A Some have voiced concern that genetic testing results may become a part of the family history and that there is potential for discrimination from the standpoint of employment and insurability. Legislation to protect against this has been discussed but whether it can be implemented effectively is unclear.

Another problem is that the majority of BRCA abnormalities are minor abnormalities that have questionable risk associated with them. The personal knowledge of carrying a very minor mutation with probably no increased risk, a mutation of undetermined significance, may cause undue anxiety with unneeded testing and even unnecessary preventative surgeries. Genetic counseling can be very helpful regarding these issues.

Q *If I have BRCA testing and it is normal, then I'm in the clear as far as inherited breast and ovarian cancer, right?*

A Unfortunately, that's not true. If you are the first one in your family to undergo BRCA testing, the result is meaningful only if the test is abnormal. This is an important point that is frequently misunderstood. Not every familial breast cancer gene is located on the current available test. There are obvious familial breast cancers with normal BRCA test results. Therefore, if your family history is very strong and you have breast cancer, despite a normal BRCA test, you may still be carrying a gene that is presently undetectable.

In high-risk families, an abnormal BRCA test has much greater significance because it confirms a hereditary breast cancer situation and other family members can subsequently undergo testing. A normal result can be falsely negative because the abnormal gene cannot be found by the current testing methods.

Having a normal test is most meaningful when someone in the family has already tested BRCA positive. Only then, if you have a normal BRCA test, can you be sure that you haven't inherited the abnormal gene.

Q *How are men affected by the BRCA gene?*

A Men who carry the gene may develop breast cancer and also may pass the gene on to their offspring. Their daughters who carry the abnormal gene will be at higher risk of breast or ovarian cancer. Whether men who carry BRCA abnormalities are at risk of other cancers is being studied actively. For men who are BRCA2 carriers, in addition to a higher risk of breast cancer, there seems to also be a higher risk of prostate cancer.

4

※

Who Should Be on My Team?

Q *Which physicians should be involved in the care of my breast cancer?*
A A breast cancer team involves a number of physicians, including a mammographer, a pathologist, a surgeon, a medical oncologist, and often a radiation oncologist. Depending on the type of breast surgery needed, sometimes a plastic surgeon is included.

Q *What does the mammographer do?*
A The mammographer is a radiologist, a physician who specializes in reading X-rays, and in particular, breast X-rays and ultrasounds. You have probably spoken with your mammographer in reviewing your mammograms because many breast cancers are first discovered by mammogram. The mammographer, using a core needle biopsy with mammogram or ultrasound guidance, now performs most breast biopsies. A mammographer is also usually the radiologist that reads breast MRIs.

Q *How does the mammographer diagnose breast cancer?*
A The diagnosis of breast cancer always relies on a biopsy. A mammogram by itself cannot diagnose cancer. In fact, up to 10 percent of all breast cancers aren't seen by mammogram. The mammographer tries

to find changes within the breast X-ray that result from breast tissue reacting to the cancer. This reaction usually results in the development of a suspicious pattern of new calcium deposits or in the formation of scar-like tissue that is different from the rest of the breast. Often an ultrasound is used to evaluate further a suspicious area. If the abnormality looks like a cyst, a benign (non-cancerous) fluid-filled cavity, it can be drained with a needle. It is very rare to have a cancer within a benign-appearing cyst. However if the abnormality appears solid, it may be suspicious for a cancer and can be biopsied with a needle.

The most informative needle biopsies are core needle biopsies. A core needle biopsy uses a hollow needle to remove a small cylinder of breast tissue. Another type of needle biopsy is an FNA, which stands for fine needle aspiration. FNA is a biopsy technique that removes only single cells. FNA biopsy is a less helpful tool when used for breast biopsy. FNA is helpful in finding breast cancer cells in lymph nodes, but within the breast, a FNA biopsy cannot distinguish between DCIS and invasive cancer. This is because the diagnosis of invasive breast cancer requires the demonstration of cancer cells invading through the duct or lobule wall, and FNA provides only singles cells without surrounding architecture. Needle biopsies of the breast should therefore be performed with core needles.

Biopsies can also be done using the mammogram through a computer-assisted device called a stereotactic core biopsy table. In this type of biopsy, a woman lies on her stomach with her breast dropping through an opening in the table. Below the table, a computer-assisted device locates the cancer and directs the biopsy needle. All state-of-the-art breast centers have this capability.

Q *Who reads the biopsy to determine that it is a cancer?*

A This is the role of the pathologist, a physician specially trained to look at biopsy specimens under the microscope. This is the only way that breast cancer can be diagnosed definitively. You should never undergo treatment for breast cancer without a biopsy that has been read by a pathologist. Many tests like a mammogram, ultrasound, or MRI can strongly suggest that a cancer is present, but only a biopsy and pathology evaluation under the microscope is considered conclusive.

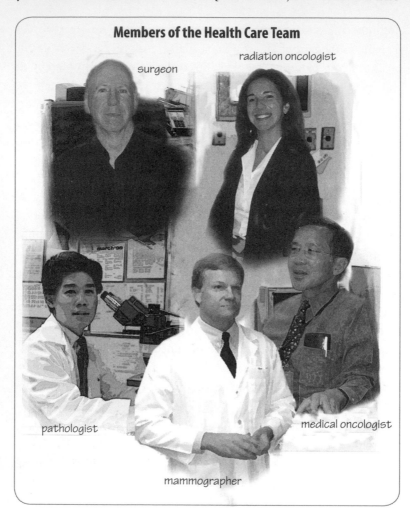

Members of the Health Care Team

surgeon

radiation oncologist

pathologist

medical oncologist

mammographer

Q *If a biopsy shows cancer, what is the next step?*

A Usually you would initially see a surgeon, although in some cases a medical oncologist is consulted first. It depends on whether the cancer is thought to be on the smaller side or is large. Smaller cancers are usually first treated with surgery, while many larger cancers are treated first with chemotherapy (or less commonly, hormonal therapy) to shrink the cancer and permit optimal surgical removal. This will be discussed in more detail in chapter 14.

Q *Should my surgeon be a breast surgeon?*

A Your surgeon should be skilled and experienced in current breast surgery techniques. You should have a surgeon who has excellent knowledge and judgment about the type of operation you need. This doesn't need to be a surgeon who only does breast surgery. Breast surgery is performed by surgeons trained initially in general surgery. The term breast surgeon can imply a surgeon who performs only breast surgery and no other type of surgery. There is presently in the United States no specialty board designation for breast surgery.

Excellent breast surgery with maximum cancer control and also excellent cosmetic results does require a high level of technical expertise. Breast surgery requires technical skill, but it isn't the most difficult surgery that most surgeons perform. Many excellent breast surgeons choose to perform other more complicated surgeries to maintain a high level of skill. This is true in community practices and also at university hospitals. Usually, physicians know who the best physicians are, and you should speak with your family physician, your mammographer, and your oncologist for a recommendation.

Q *When do I need to see a plastic surgeon?*

A If you need to have a mastectomy, a consultation with a plastic surgeon will help you learn about your options for breast reconstruction. These options are reviewed in chapter 8. If you are interested in breast reconstruction, having the reconstruction done at the same time as mastectomy can give a better cosmetic result. This is not always possible, particularly if it is thought that you might need radiation after mastectomy.

Q *If I need to see a medical oncologist first, is that bad?*

A No, it's not necessarily bad. Although it's certainly more advantageous to have a smaller cancer rather than a larger one, some patients have a small cancer but also have a small breast size. If this is the case in your situation, you have a better chance of avoiding a mastectomy if the cancer can be reduced in size before surgery. Patients with larger cancers who require chemotherapy before surgery can also have a very good outcome as a result of effective treatment.

Q *Should the medical oncologist be a breast specialist?*

A The medical oncologist should be experienced and knowledgeable in treating breast cancer. Because breast cancer is the most common major cancer in women in North America, the treatment of breast cancer comprises a large portion of a medical oncologist's training and practice. In North America there are no specific breast cancer training programs or board certification for the sole purpose of treating breast cancer.

Your oncologist should be skilled in the treatment of breast cancer but does not necessarily have to have a practice limited to breast cancer. Your primary care physician, mammographer, and surgeon should be able to guide you in selecting an excellent oncologist and you can also contact your local university breast center for a referral.

Q *Who should be leading my team?*

A The medical oncologist usually leads the team. However, if the cancer is on the smaller side, initial surgery is often performed prior to an evaluation with a medical oncologist because lumpectomy and sentinel node biopsy is routinely recommended first. This doesn't mean that your oncologist did not have input on the type of surgery you need. Many quality breast cancer treatment programs have a weekly breast cancer meeting where all new breast cancer patients are reviewed and treatment strategy is discussed. The mammogram, ultrasound, and biopsy are studied by the physicians. Then the surgeons, radiation oncologists, and medical oncologists discuss the best treatment strategy for each patient. You should ask if your case has been reviewed in this manner.

THE BREAST CANCER team is meeting at the weekly hospital breast conference to review all of the new breast cancer patients. Those present include a mammographer, pathologists, surgeons, medical oncologists, and radiation oncologists.

The mammographer, Dr. Calipari, begins by showing each patient's mammograms and ultrasounds projected on a large screen. Using a laser pointer to highlight the abnormalities, she begins, "This is a seventy-seven year-old (the patient is always assumed to be female unless otherwise specified) with a 1.5 cm abnormal calcification in the lower outer quadrant of the left breast. It's non-palpable (can't be felt). Ultrasound shows a 2.2 cm mass in the same area and the axilla is clear (no abnormal nodes on ultrasound)."

Next the pathologist, Dr. Klass, projects the images of the biopsy on to the screen. "This is an invasive ductal carcinoma, grade 2 with associated high-grade DCIS. ER is 80 percent, PR is 40 percent, Her2 is negative, and Ki-67 is 10 percent."

One of the surgeons, Dr. Silver, begins the discussion, "Well, the patient is seventy-seven, judging by the mammos she has fairly small breasts, maybe a B cup. The simplest approach is probably a mastectomy and sentinel node biopsy, unless she really wants to save her breast."

Katie, the nurse practitioner from the breast center, interjects, "I spoke with her yesterday and she's very energetic and spry. She's a widow but came with her boyfriend who's been with her for about a year. I reviewed with her the options for surgery and if possible, she'd definitely like to save her breast."

Dr. Silver replies, "Well, then let's have Dr. Calipari bracket the calcifications and we'll excise between the wires and see what kind of cosmetic results we get."

I turn to one of the radiation oncologists, Dr. Todd, and ask, "If we get margins, you'll go ahead with radiation?" He nods his head in the affirmative. I then add, "And we'll also give her an AI (aromatase inhibitor) for five years."

As a result of this type of conference, the breast cancer team has a working plan prior to seeing and examining the patient, which will usually occur with individual separate consultations with surgeon, medical oncologist, and radiation oncologist. Of course, plans may change after actually speaking with a patient and examining her, but it's a good way to begin the decision-making process.

Q *Do I need to see a radiation oncologist?*

A Not all patients need to see a radiation oncologist. Certainly all patients with invasive cancer, and most patients with DCIS undergoing breast conservation instead of mastectomy need to be considered for radiation therapy following lumpectomy. Some patients who have mastectomy also need radiation afterward for situations where the cancer is large or where there is involvement of multiple lymph nodes. Radiation therapy is almost always given after breast surgery, not before.

Q *Do I still need to see my primary care physician?*

A Yes. Even though you have breast cancer, the chances are good that you will do well. Therefore, it is important for you to not ignore other medical problems and to continue good general medical care to optimize your health.

5

What Is Breast Imaging?

Q *How does a mammogram work?*

A A mammogram uses conventional X-rays to image the breast. During the X-ray, the breast needs to be squeezed or compressed to permit a clearer picture. This is often uncomfortable but is very necessary to achieve the best image of your breast.

Q *Where should I get a mammogram?*

A A number of studies show that centers and mammographers that perform the most mammograms, not surprisingly, also read them the most accurately and miss the smallest number of cancers. So it's not a bad thing to call to schedule a routine mammogram and be told that there is a waiting period of several months. Of course, if the mammogram is not routine but is being done to evaluate a breast lump, getting an appointment within two weeks is very important.

DR. PATRICIA JONES is an experienced and confident mammographer. She can read 70 to 90 mammograms a day, both quickly and expertly. As she reviews with me the mammograms of a patient with a new breast

American Cancer Society Guidelines for Early Detection of Breast Cancer

Women at Average Risk

Begin mammography at age 40

For women in their 20s and 30s, it is recommended that clinical breast examination be part of a periodic health examination, preferably at least every three years. Asymptomatic women aged 40 and over should continue to receive a clinical breast examination as part of a periodic health examination, preferably annually.

Beginning in their 20s, women should be told about the benefits and limitations of breast self-examination (BSE). The importance of prompt reporting of any new breast symptoms to a health professional should be emphasized. Women who choose to do BSE should receive instruction and have their technique reviewed on the occasion of a periodic health examination. It is acceptable for women to choose not to do BSE or to do BSE irregularly.

Women should have an opportunity to become informed about the benefits, limitations, and potential harms associated with regular screening.

Older Women

Screening decisions in older women should be individualized by considering the potential benefits and risks of mammography in the context of current health status and estimated life expectancy. As long as a woman is in reasonably good health and would be a candidate for treatment, she should continue to be screened with mammography.

Women at Increased Risk

Women at increased risk of breast cancer might benefit from additional screening strategies beyond those offered to women of average risk, such as earlier initiation of screening, shorter screening intervals, or the addition of screening modalities other than mammography and physical examination, such as ultrasound or magnetic resonance imaging. However, the evidence currently available is insufficient to justify recommendations of any of these screening approaches.

American Cancer Society 2003 Breast Cancer Detection Guidelines cancer, I remark, "I need a lot of time to look at a mammogram and even then often only pick up the abnormality because you've circled it with a red pencil. It's amazing how you can do it so fast."

She takes her eyes away from the films and peers at me over her reading glasses, like a professor teaching a student. She explains crisply, "It's pattern recognition and having a trained eye. If I asked you to find a dime in a fistful of other coins, you could do it very quickly after spreading the coins out on a table and glancing at them. You wouldn't have to pick up each coin, turn it over and study each one individually, trying to decide which were dimes. You could do it in a couple of seconds. It's kind of like that."

Q *Can a breast cancer be missed on a mammogram?*

A Unfortunately yes. Up to 10 percent of all breast cancers will not show up on a mammogram. At present the smallest cancer that can be detected is about 2 to 3 millimeters. One millimeter is about the width of a line drawn with a sharp pencil. However, most breast cancers cannot be seen at that small size because in many women the breasts are too dense and small abnormalities are not visible. A denser breast is harder to read and younger premenopausal women tend to have denser breasts compared to older postmenopausal women. Breast density decreases significantly with age and with menopause. As I discussed, the mammogram is not detecting the cancer itself but instead detects a change in breast tissue as a reaction to the cancer. This is usually either the deposit of abnormal patterns of calcium or the development of scar tissue. If the breast doesn't have these types of reaction to the cancer, the cancer cannot be detected at a small size.

Q *I'm disappointed and upset because when I look at my mammogram from last year that was read as normal, I can see the cancer there. Was my mammogram misread?*

A This is a surprisingly frequent question. Mammograms are sometimes difficult to read because some women, particularly younger premenopausal women, have dense breasts on mammogram. This means that the image on X-ray is very cloudy and small abnormalities can't be easily seen. It's very easy to read a mammogram when you know where the cancer is. It's not unlike finding a needle in a haystack after someone points it out to you. A mammogram always has small irregularities due to normal differences in breast tissue. It's not uncommon to be able to go back and point to one of these irregularities and say that that was your breast cancer one or two years ago. This does not mean that those mammograms were misread. More often than not, if you take those mammograms to another mammographer and have them read without knowledge of your breast cancer, they will again be read as normal.

THIS IS NATALIE'S second visit with me. She is forty-six, has four children, and owns a small retail women's clothing store. She and Mark, her husband, have questions for me prior to her upcoming surgery. She has her mammograms in hand and says, "Dr. Chan, I'm upset that they didn't find the cancer last year. When I went for a second opinion, the doctor showed me the cancer on my mammogram and then he pointed out that it was also there last year, just smaller. Did they make a mistake reading my mammogram last year?" Both she and her husband appear worried and angry.

I place her mammograms on a view-box for them to see. Her current breast cancer is circled in red, a larger denser cloud among other smaller clouds. I check her previous mammogram from last year and can now see the smaller cloud from among other small clouds that a year later turned out to be the current cancer. However one year ago, that spot didn't really look much different than any other. Only in hindsight is it obvious. I point this out to Natalie and Mark, and as they study the mammograms, they can see how difficult it would have been to call this spot abnormal last year.

"Look, you've got four kids. Do any of them read those *Where's Waldo* books, the ones where Waldo is hidden within a very complex drawing?" She nods her head. "You know how hard it is for the kids to find him. They have to look a long time. But once they've found him, when they know where he is, they can find him quickly after that. Well it's similar to looking at previous mammograms or previous scans of any kind. When you know where the problem is, you can always go back to the earlier picture and see where it started. That doesn't mean that the earlier picture actually shows an abnormality."

They nod in understanding, noticeably less upset. We can now move on to dealing with the current problem.

Q *I've heard that some studies show that mammograms do not save lives.*
A Like many things in medicine, there are some conflicting studies about mammograms. A few studies seem to show that lives aren't saved by mammograms, while other studies clearly demonstrate that mammograms taken with high quality equipment and read by well-trained mammographers are effective in saving lives. At the present time, there isn't a better screening method. Options may change as MRI and other techniques develop over the next several years.

Results of the Breast Cancer Screening Trials on Breast Cancer Mortality Reduction

Study	Age Range	% Mortality Reduction (95% CI)	
HIP	40–64	24%	(7, 38)
Malmö	45–69	19%	(-8, 39)
Two-County Trial, Sweden	40–75	32%	(20, 41)
Edinburgh	45–64	21%	(-2, 40)
Stockholm	40–64	26%	(-10, 50)
Canada NBSS-1	40–49	-3%	(-26, 27)
Canada NBSS-2	50–59	-2%	(-33 22)
Gothenburg	39–59*	16%	(-39, 49)
All Trials Combined	**39–75**	**24%**	**(18, 30)**

Reference: American Cancer Society

Having mammograms saves lives as demonstrated by this table of studies which show an overall reduction in death by 24%.

Mammogram

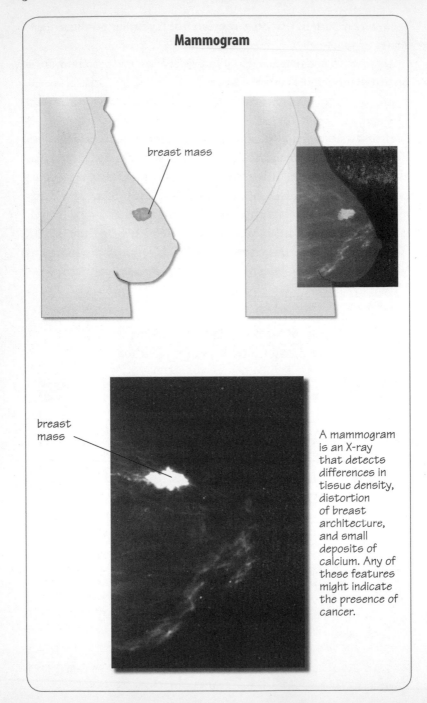

breast mass

breast mass

A mammogram is an X-ray that detects differences in tissue density, distortion of breast architecture, and small deposits of calcium. Any of these features might indicate the presence of cancer.

Q *How can I know that I'm receiving good quality mammograms?*

A You need to go to a dedicated breast-imaging center that does a large number of mammograms. Usually this is a center where a routine mammogram may take over one to two months to schedule. The mammotech (technician who performs the mammogram) should spend some time making sure that your breast is squeezed properly to achieve a clear picture. There should be a full-time mammographer always present to review the films. Optimally, the mammograms would be double read, either by two mammographers or checked by using a computer assisted software program called CAD.

Q *What about ultrasound?*

A Ultrasound of the breast uses radar-like technology to generate images, as sound waves travel through the breast tissue. Ultrasound of the breast can be a helpful tool, but is most helpful when a specific area of the breast can be targeted. This is because ultrasound imaging requires some technical manipulation and it is difficult to have a high quality ultrasound of the entire breast with currently existing equipment. Therefore ultrasound is most helpful in evaluating a specific suspicious area on mammogram or a lump that can be felt within the breast. As advances in ultrasound technique and equipment occur, that may change and ultrasound may become a more frequently used screening tool, rather than a test that is most useful for targeting a specific spot within the breast.

Q *What is MRI of the breast?*

A MRI stands for magnetic resonance imaging. It's another way to try to obtain an internal picture of the body by using a computer to generate a picture using differences in electromagnetic fields produced by different tissues. This is a very promising imaging tool for breast cancer but is also very new, somewhat difficult to interpret, and very expensive. Although MRI of other organs has been used for years, MRI of the breast has become widely available only since 2003. This newness in breast MRI has resulted in certain problems. The software for generating high quality pictures is still under development and images can differ significantly from one machine to another.

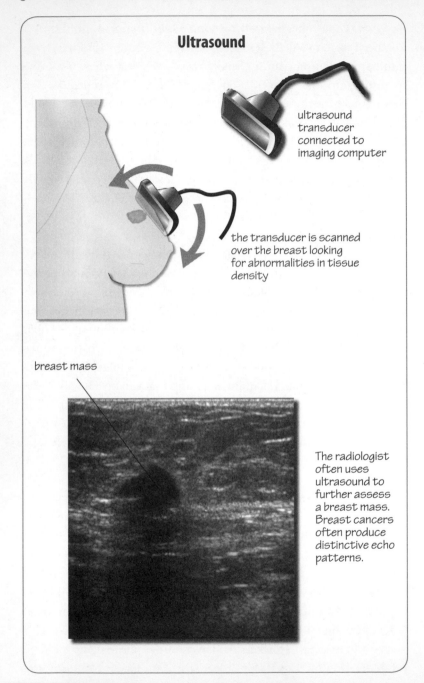

Ultrasound

ultrasound transducer connected to imaging computer

the transducer is scanned over the breast looking for abnormalities in tissue density

breast mass

The radiologist often uses ultrasound to further assess a breast mass. Breast cancers often produce distinctive echo patterns.

A major problem is the current lack of uniformity in reading and interpreting a breast MRI. Mammographers have national guidelines that are clearly established for reading a mammogram. It is required that reported findings on a mammogram for *normal* and *abnormal* conform to these national standards. Because MRI of the breast is very new, at this time there are no clear guidelines on what findings constitute *normal* and *abnormal*.

Unlike mammogram and ultrasound, breast MRI involves the injection of a contrast agent into the vein. The contrast helps illuminate abnormalities within the breast and can result in the detection of many small abnormalities, many of which aren't cancers. This is a significant potential problem. That is why Dr. Laura Liberman, a national expert in this field from Memorial Sloan-Kettering Cancer Center in New York, doesn't feel (summer 2004) that MRI is ready for routine breast screening, because it may lead to excessive and unnecessary biopsies of non-cancerous MRI abnormalities. That of course may change as more and more studies of MRI breast screening are reported and the technique improves.

There are now some studies showing that MRI is a good screening tool for women who carry the BRCA gene abnormality. This seems to be because their chances of having breast cancer are much higher, and therefore if an abnormality is found on MRI, there is a greater chance that the abnormality is due to breast cancer than if it were found on an MRI of a woman who is BRCA negative.

Q *Who should be having a breast MRI?*

A In September 2004, the American Society of Breast Surgeons published a consensus statement regarding when breast MRI should be used. The recommendations make sense and essentially summarize common use today. They suggest MRI as a screening test only in women with very high risk of breast cancer such as those with BRCA mutations. They also recommend MRI in patients with known breast cancer when the size or exact location of the cancer is difficult to determine on mammogram. This frequently happens with invasive lobular cancer where mammogram images can underestimate the

Magnetic Resonance Imaging (MRI)

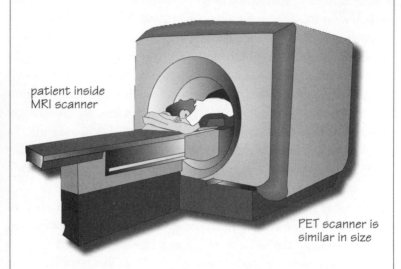

patient inside
MRI scanner

PET scanner is
similar in size

breast cancer

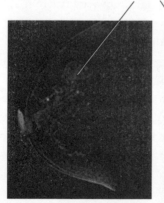
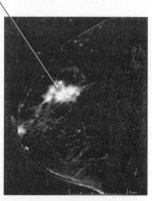

MRI with and without contrast

actual cancer size. MRI may also be helpful for some women who have mammogram and ultrasounds that are difficult to read for technical reasons.

Q *Are PET scans being used to image breast cancer?*

A A PET scan is a scan that uses a computer to generate an image of a body part based on the difference in uptake of blood sugar between normal and abnormal tissue. PET stands for positron emission tomography. At first it was hoped that PET would be a perfect test for cancer because cancers take up sugar from the blood at a faster rate than normal tissues. Unfortunately, it turns out that areas of infection and inflammation are also abnormal by PET, making interpretation less certain. Experience shows that PET often cannot see cancers that are less than 10 mm, so many small cancers can be missed on PET. Unfortunately, like other tests used in cancer detection, PET will miss small cancers and not every abnormality will necessarily be a cancer. At the present time, PET screening of the breast is primarily a research tool, although it can be an excellent test when used appropriately in other cancer situations. Currently PET is used more effectively to stage and detect spreading breast cancer to other body areas.

Q *I've heard a lot recently about ductal lavage. What is it?*

A Ductal lavage has been studied extensively over the past several years. A prominent breast surgeon, Dr. Susan Love, brought it to national attention as a possible way of detecting a breast cancer early. The way this test works is that a very small tube is inserted into the duct system via the nipple. Unfortunately, for some women this can be painful. Fluid is forced into the duct and then withdrawn and analyzed to see if cancer cells are present. If cancer cells are found in the fluid specimen, the test doesn't tell you where in the duct system the cancer is. Nevertheless, at first, this seemed like a very promising test. However, recent studies of ductal lavage in women who have biopsy-proven breast cancer show a disappointingly low chance of detecting cancer cells by ductal lavage. If other studies confirm a low percentage detection rate of cancer, ductal lavage will not be considered a helpful diagnostic tool.

Positron Emission Tomography (PET) Scan

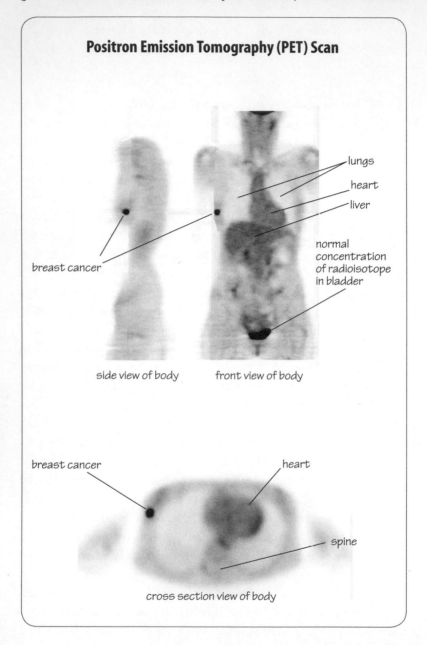

side view of body   front view of body

cross section view of body

6

❊

What Do I Need to Know about My Pathology Report?

Q *What is a pathology report?*

A It is absolutely essential for breast cancer to be diagnosed by biopsy. Although mammograms and ultrasounds may be very suspicious, only a biopsy can unequivocally confirm the diagnosis of breast cancer. A pathology report is the report generated by a physician called a pathologist who examines the biopsy specimen by using a microscope. The biopsy material is fixed in wax, then cut very thinly and placed on microscope slides. The slides are stained to give color contrast to the different cells. Then they are examined with a microscope. The process of preparing and reading a slide generally takes at least one to two days.

Every time a biopsy or surgery is performed, the specimen is tested this way and a pathology report is generated. For most breast cancer patients, there will be two reports. The first report is for the initial breast biopsy. A second or final report is made after definitive breast surgery.

Typical Pathology Report

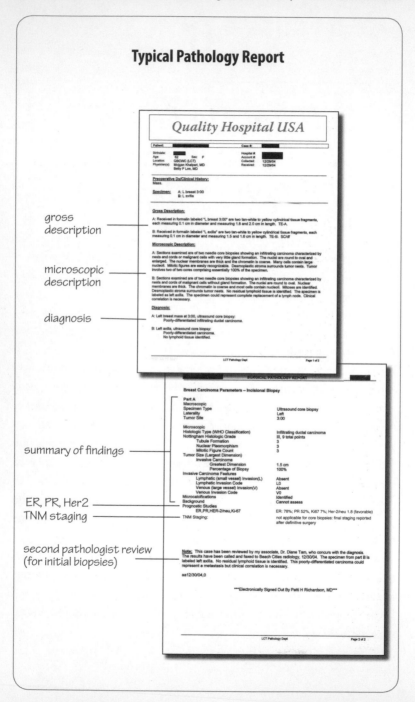

gross description

microscopic description

diagnosis

summary of findings

ER, PR, Her2
TNM staging

second pathologist review
(for initial biopsies)

Q *What should be in the report?*

A The most basic part of the report should state whether or not cancer is present, what type of cancer it is, and whether the cancer is invasive or in situ (noninvasive). The pathologist will also assign a grade to the cancer; low, intermediate, or high. The grade is a comment on the potential aggressive behavior of the cancer based upon certain characteristics that can be observed under the microscope. If the biopsy is performed using a needle, it is not possible to estimate the size of the cancer by biopsy alone.

I STOP BY the pathology office after my hospital rounds, before heading to the office. My assistant had paged a message to me that a soon-to-be-seen new patient, Mrs. Jackson, does not yet have a printed pathology report for me to review and so I've come to pathology to find out why. The secretary informs me that Dr. Ross is the pathologist in charge of Mrs. Jackson's case.

He's examining a slide with his microscope as I interrupt and ask, "Hey Tom, what's the hang-up on the path report on Jackson? I thought we reviewed it at breast conference."

Looking up from his work, he replies, "Hi, Dave. I know at the conference I said she had ADH, but one of the other pathologists also looked at her slides and he thinks that there may also be DCIS. You know we always have more than one set of eyes looking at this stuff. So there's no report yet because we've sent the slides out for a second opinion with Page at Vanderbilt. It'll probably take four to five days."

I'm always impressed by how careful the physicians are to make the right call and to check their work. Mammographers often ask patients to come back for additional views or ultrasound because they think that they see something. More often than not, these "callbacks" are normal. By the same token, the pathologists I work with always show their cases to colleagues to confirm that the biopsy is being read correctly.

All difficult cancer cases are reviewed at Tumor Board or discussed informally among associates or sent for second opinions to make sure that the correct treatment plan is in place. Everyone tries to do his or her best for each patient.

---

should be on the report?

...omarker analysis should be performed on all invasive cancers, and in a more limited extent, also on DCIS. This type of evaluation tests each patient's cancer cells directly. The testing should include analysis for the presence or absence of receptors for estrogen and progesterone. This is often referred to as ER and PR for estrogen receptor and progesterone receptor. The specimen is also tested for a gene mutation called Her2. Lastly, an estimation of cancer growth rate can be measured by Ki-67.

Q *What is the significance of ER and PR?*

A If the breast cancer is ER or PR positive, the likelihood is increased that the cancer will respond to hormone therapy that uses a number of different drugs to alter estrogen level or estrogen activity within the body. This will be discussed in more detail in chapter 12. Cancers that are ER and PR positive have these receptors on the cells and seem to use estrogen to grow. ER and PR positive cancers tend to grow more slowly and have a weaker tendency to spread to lymph nodes. ER and PR are reported as the percentage of cells that stain for the receptor. With the use of a microscope, the stains reveal the presence of the receptors. The higher the number, the more likely the breast cancer needs hormones to grow and spread, and therefore the more likely the cancer is to respond to hormonal therapies.

Q *What is the significance of Her2?*

A Her2 is an oncogene, a non-inherited gene mutation that occurs in up to 20 to 25 percent of breast cancers. Oncogenes are important in that they control growth and spread of cancer. The relationship between Her2 and breast cancer was discovered by Dr. Dennis Slamon at UCLA. Breast cancers that contain the Her2 mutation are called Her2 positive. Her2 positive breast cancers tend to grow faster and have a greater tendency to spread.

The most common way to test for Her2 is with a test called IHC, but the more accurate (and more expensive and labor intensive) test technique is called FISH (fluorescence in situ hybridization). Her2 analysis by FISH is not usually included in most standard pathology lab analysis and therefore may need to be ordered separately if the Her2 status will influence a treatment decision. Your oncologist will be aware of this and order the FISH test if needed. There is also a treatment, similar to hormonal therapy targeting hormone receptors, that specifically targets Her2 called Herceptin. I'll discuss this further in chapter 13.

Q *Why is the growth rate important and how is this measured?*
A Ki-67 is currently considered the most reliable way of estimating how fast the breast cancer grows. Faster growing cancers tend to also have higher potential to spread to other areas of the body. Ki-67 is a test that detects a protein that is important in cell growth in the nucleus of the cancer cells. If a cell is about to divide, there is a lot of this protein present within the nucleus and this can be seen by a special staining technique with a microscope. Having more than 10 percent of cells with Ki-67 staining is considered elevated. The higher the number, the greater the growth rate of the cancer. Very fast-growing breast cancers can have Ki-67 levels of 60 to 80 percent, indicating that 60 to 80 percent of the cells are preparing to divide.

Q *Why are the biomarkers significant?*
A Biomarkers discussed above are important because they're unique characteristics of your specific breast cancer. The results of your biomarkers will often be used to help determine if you need adjuvant therapy and what type of therapy you should receive. Your cancer's biomarkers can be used to help provide an estimate of your chances of having a recurrence. The use of specific treatments such as hormonal therapies and Herceptin are based upon having the appropriate biomarkers that indicate whether or not the treatments might be effective for you. For example if you are ER and PR negative, hormone therapy would not be expected to be helpful in reducing recurrence risk for you.

   If you are Her2 negative, Herceptin would not be effective and shouldn't be included as part of your treatment.

Breast Markers Used by Pathologists

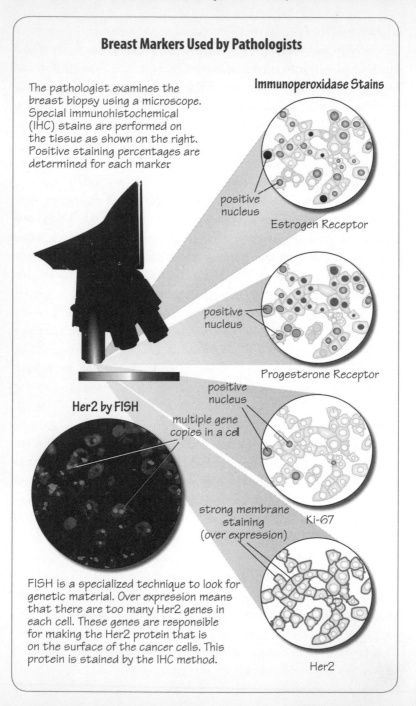

The pathologist examines the breast biopsy using a microscope. Special immunohistochemical (IHC) stains are performed on the tissue as shown on the right. Positive staining percentages are determined for each marker

Immunoperoxidase Stains

positive nucleus

Estrogen Receptor

positive nucleus

Progesterone Receptor

positive nucleus

Ki-67

Her2 by FISH

multiple gene copies in a cell

strong membrane staining (over expression)

Her2

FISH is a specialized technique to look for genetic material. Over expression means that there are too many Her2 genes in each cell. These genes are responsible for making the Her2 protein that is on the surface of the cancer cells. This protein is stained by the IHC method.

Q *What is the Oncotype DX Breast Cancer Assay?*

A This is a new commercially available test of gene expression (activity) in breast cancer tissue. The test uses a technique called PCR, which is polymerase chain reaction, to measure messenger RNA that is produced by the DNA activity. In other words, the test can measure minute amounts of material made by certain genes important in breast cancer growth. This test is an analysis of the activity of a panel of twenty-one genes that researchers consider important in predicting breast cancer behavior. The analysis is performed on the biopsy tissue and attempts to separate breast cancer patients into three groups with respect to risk of relapse; low, intermediate, and high. Of significance is that the genes whose activities are considered most important are the genes that control hormone receptors, Her2, and proliferative rate. These are already reported in other testing methods, as discussed above, but this test helps confirm the validity of the factors that oncologists have traditionally used to estimate recurrence risk.

Whether Oncotype DX will be a more accurate measurement of biologic activity will depend on the results of further studies. For now, however, this test may be considered for patients who are lymph node negative and hormone receptor positive, but are borderline for chemotherapy because of other factors. The test needs to be specially ordered and is also very expensive, about $3,500. It's important to note that Oncotype DX has been evaluated only in patients who are lymph node negative. This is the first of many tests to come that will attempt to analyze directly the genetic profile of a breast cancer in an attempt to predict its behavior. In the future, oncologists may use this kind of information to select the most appropriate treatment. For now, the benefit of this test is not yet proven.

Q *What is gene microarray technology?*

A This is a technique that uses the so-called gene chip technology to analyze all the genetic material in any cell, including cancer cells. Over 30,000 genes can be analyzed on a single chip. The gene chip creates a genetic profile of the cancer. Early studies indicate that this profiling may be helpful in determining what chemotherapies should be used in treating each specific cancer. These tests aren't yet commercially available, but are being studied in a number of important clinical trials. Oncologists are hopeful that this test will greatly assist in chemotherapy selection. We are currently testing gene microarray to try to predict response to preoperative chemotherapy in a study directed by Dr. Helena Chang at UCLA.

Q *What is the final pathology report?*

A The final pathology report usually refers to the report completed by the pathologist following breast surgery when all the material has been thoroughly examined and testing is complete. The essential information should include the final size of the breast cancer, whether or not it has gone into lymph nodes, the number of lymph nodes involved, and the extent of cancer in each node. There should be a comment on the margins of the surgery and whether or not the cancer had been completely excised. If the cancer contains both an invasive portion and a noninvasive portion (DCIS), there should be a measurement of the size of each component. The cancer cells are also analyzed under the microscope for degree of differentiation, that is, how closely the cancer resembles normal breast cells. This is often reported on a numeric scale called ScharfBloomRichardson, with the higher numbers indicating a greater tendency for aggressive behavior. There should also be a comment on whether or not cancer cells are present in lymphatic or blood vessel spaces within the breast (lymphovascular invasion).

Most breast cancer programs will have this essential information listed in a table format, which will help your physicians decide on the best treatment for your particular situation. The form would also include a TNM stage at the end of the report. The biomarkers will often be included in this report or can be reported separately. This report, which organizes all existing data about your breast cancer, helps your team of physicians decide whether any additional surgery is required, and also whether chemotherapy, hormonal therapy, or radiation therapy is needed.

Q *What is the TNM stage that my report refers to?*

A This is a kind of shorthand your physicians use to reflect how much cancer there is for each individual patient. The T stage refers to the

Breast Cancer TNM Staging

Stage	T Stage Size of Cancer	Metastatic Cancer Cells In:	
		N Stage Lymph Nodes	M Stage Other Organs
0	**Tis:** any size (carcinoma in situ)	**N0:** no	**M0:** no
I	**T1:** small (less than 2 cm)	**N0:** no	**M0:** no
IIA	**T1:** small (less than 2 cm)	**N1:** yes	**M0:** no
	T2: medium (2 cm-5 cm)	**N0:** no	**M0:** no
	T0: no cancer is found in breast	**N1:** yes	**M0:** no
IIB	**T2:** medium (2 cm-5 cm)	**N1:** yes	**M0:** no
	T3: large (>5 cm)	**N0:** no	**M0:** no
IIIA	**T1:** small (less than 2 cm)	**N2:** yes	**M0:** no
	T2: medium (2 cm-5 cm)	**N2:** yes	**M0:** no
	T3: large (>5 cm)	**N1:** yes	**M0:** no
	T3: large (>5 cm)	**N2:** yes	**M0:** no
	T0: no cancer is found in breast	**N2:** yes	**M0:** no
IIIB	**T4:** any size but spread to chest wall or skin (inflammatory carcinoma)	**N0, 1, 2, or 3:** yes or no	**M0:** no
IIIC	**T1, 2 or 3:** any size	**N3:** yes	**M0:** no
IV	**T1, 2 or 3:** any size	**N0, 1, 2, or 3:** yes or no	**M1:** yes

N 1:   breast cancer cells in 1-3 axillary lymph nodes

N 2:   breast cancer cells in 4-9 axillary nine lymph and the lymph nodes are also enlarged, and/or attached to each other or to nearby tissue or
1 or more internal mammary lymph nodes (under sternum) which are not enlarged (cancer seen only under the microscope) but not in any axillary lymph nodes

N 3:   breast cancer cells in 10 or more axillary lymph nodes or
1 or more lymph nodes above or below the collarbone (infraclavicular or supraclavicular nodes) or
1 or more enlarged internal mammary lymph nodes (all nodes are on the same side as the breast cancer)

TX, NX, or MX: tumor, lymph node, or distant spread to organs cannot be assessed size of the invasive component of your breast cancer. The T will have a number next to it and a letter modifier. The higher numbers and letters indicate a larger size cancer. For example a T1a cancer is less than 0.5 cm, while a T1b is greater than 0.5 cm but less than 1.0 cm. A T2 cancer is 2 to 5 cm in size. The N stage refers to the lymph node status. If the lymph nodes are free of cancer, the N will have a zero next to it. The higher the N number, the more lymph nodes involved. The M stage refers to the status of having metastatic disease outside of the breast and lymph nodes. An M with a zero next to it indicates that there is no evidence that the cancer has spread to other areas of the body.

During clinical trials when there are head-to-head comparisons of different treatments, the TNM staging system is very helpful in assisting researchers to make sure that similar groups of patients are being studied. The TNM staging is also very helpful to your oncologist in placing your cancer within a specific risk group to allow proper selection of adjuvant treatments as will be discussed in chapters 11, 12, and 13. The higher the TNM stage, the lower the chance that surgery alone will cure the cancer. Higher TNM stage cancers tend to require more treatments to achieve a cure.

7

❋

What Are My Options for Breast Treatment?

Q *I have been told I have breast cancer. Which physician should I see first?*
A After diagnosis of breast cancer, patients will usually see a surgeon first because for most patients, breast surgery will be the first treatment. If the cancer is larger than average, you may also be seeing an oncologist prior to surgery for consideration of pre-operative chemotherapy.

Q *Whom do I see for breast surgery? Do I need to see a breast surgeon?*
A I would recommend that you see a surgeon who is experienced in breast surgery, has sound judgment regarding the type of surgery needed, and has superior technical skill in breast surgery. As previously discussed, there is no specialty board designation for breast surgery. A good way to start is by speaking with your family physician and your mammographer for a referral. As an oncologist with over twenty years experience in treating breast cancer, I've seen the results of many breast surgeries performed by a wide range of surgeons. In my experience, the best results seem to come from surgeons who are technically skilled and maintain their high level of surgical precision by also performing a variety of challenging non-breast-cancer operations. However there

are also excellent surgeons who limit their practice to breast surgery only. Your oncologist can also help you make a selection.

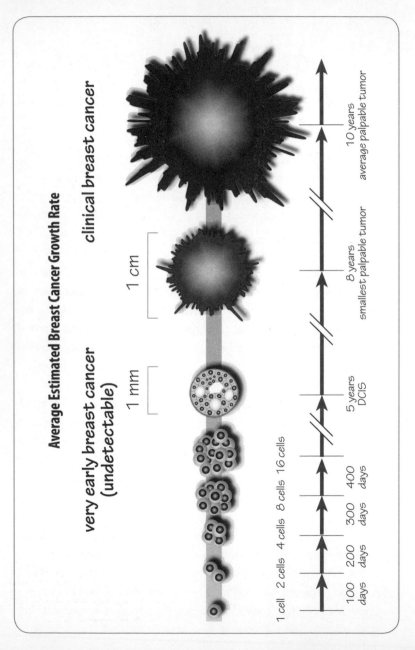

Average Estimated Breast Cancer Growth Rate

very early breast cancer (undetectable)   *clinical breast cancer*

1 mm   1 cm

1 cell   2 cells   4 cells   8 cells   16 cells

100 days   200 days   300 days   400 days   5 years DCIS   8 years smallest palpable tumor   10 years average palpable tumor

The surgeons that I work with in the community and the breast surgeons currently at UCLA perform breast surgery as one part of a portfolio of many operations. From the standpoint of technical skill, there may be an advantage when breast surgery is not the most difficult surgery that the surgeon performs. The counterpoint to this argument, of course, is that your surgeon should be experienced in breast surgery and that doing something often is a great advantage in perfecting technique. It's not unreasonable to ask your surgeon how many breast surgeries he or she has performed.

Q *Is breast surgery an emergency? Should I have it right away?*

A No, there's no need to rush. Many studies have shown that, based on the growth rate of the average breast cancer, the time taken to grow from the initial single cancer cell to a cancer 1 cm in diameter is about six to eight years. Therefore, for the average patient with breast cancer, having surgery performed within a time frame of two months is reasonable. This permits time for second opinions, a careful and thoughtful decision on the best surgical approach, selection of a surgeon that you are comfortable with and have confidence in, and for completing important personal commitments such as making arrangements for coverage at work, taking a scheduled vacation, or attending your child's wedding.

Q *What is a lumpectomy?*

A A lumpectomy is surgical removal of an area of breast tissue that encompasses the entire cancer. This is also sometimes called a partial mastectomy or segmental mastectomy. Mastectomy refers to removal of breast tissue and the words partial or segmental indicate that the removal is not removal of the entire breast. The goal of lumpectomy is complete removal of the cancer with a surrounding border of normal breast tissue. This permits radiation to save or conserve the breast (also known as breast conservation) and results in the lowest chance of recurrence within the breast. The area of breast removed is typically not round but more like removal of a wedge of an orange with the goal of capturing the cancer within the center of the wedge. This permits minimal disruption of the normal shape of the breast and gives the best appearance afterward. The best incisions aren't straight but curved and loosely follow the natural curve of the breast and the curve of the areola (the colored area around the nipple).

Q *When is a lumpectomy performed?*

A The purpose of a lumpectomy is to permit breast conservation by avoiding the need to remove the breast completely (a mastectomy). Healing from the surgery usually takes about three to four weeks. Usually you are comfortable and not incapacitated, although it is not advised that you go to work or even do light exercise for ten to fourteen days. For

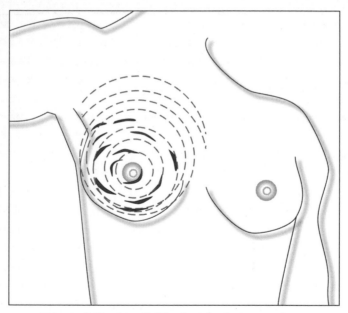

Recommended Locations of Incisions for Lumpectomy

Recommended locations of incisions for performing lumpectomy are shown in the above illustration. For large lesions in the lower breast, particularly when skin must be excisied, a radial incision often results in better cosmesis. *Adapted from Bland KI and Copeland EM (eds.).* The Breast: Comprehensive Management of Benign and Malignant Diseases. *Philadelphia. PA: WB Saunders; 1998; 802-816.*

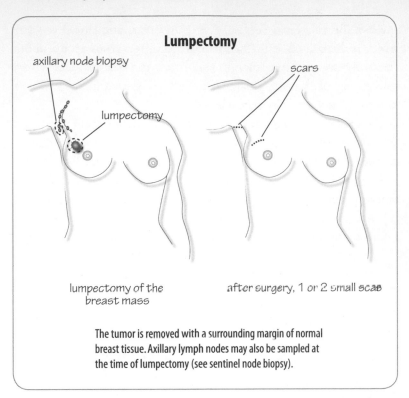

Lumpectomy

axillary node biopsy

scars

lumpectomy

lumpectomy of the
breast mass

after surgery, 1 or 2 small scars

The tumor is removed with a surrounding margin of normal
breast tissue. Axillary lymph nodes may also be sampled at
the time of lumpectomy (see sentinel node biopsy).

the large majority of patients with invasive breast cancer, radiation
therapy is required after the lumpectomy has healed. For patients with
DCIS that is small and low grade, sometimes radiation is omitted,
but this is controversial and will be discussed in chapter 10.

Q *What is meant by the margins of resection and why is this important?*
A Achieving clear margins is essential for having a successful lumpectomy.
The outside edges of the lumpectomy are called the margins and they
need to be completely free of cancer. Among experts there is some
debate over exactly how much margin is optimal before radiation
can be given for breast conservation. Studies indicate that if there are
cancer cells at the margin, the rate of cancer recurrence within the
breast may be 20 to 25 percent, which is not acceptable. For invasive
breast cancer, the minimum requirement is no cancer cells visible at
the margins of the lumpectomy and that is the criteria required by

the NSABP (National Surgical Adjuvant Breast and Bowel Project), which is the United States' national breast cancer study group. Some specialists want a larger margin than that, and desire at least 2 to 3 millimeters of clear margin, a millimeter being roughly the width of a line drawn with a sharp pencil.

For DCIS, the margins need to be somewhat larger because the cancer cells are only in the ducts and the duct system is serpentine, winding in and out of otherwise normal breast tissue. In DCIS, the minimal margin is generally having at least one normal duct between the DCIS and the margin. Therefore the margins for DCIS need to be more generous than the margins for invasive cancer. This at first seems paradoxical because DCIS is considered a less serious problem. However, it makes sense

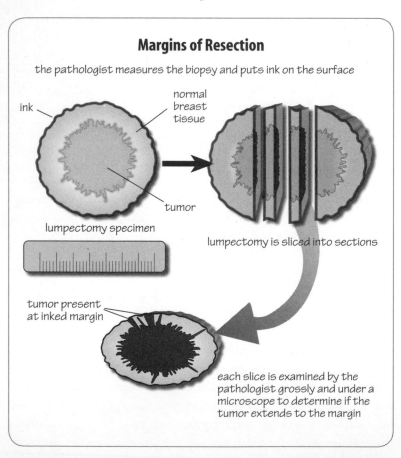

Margins of Resection

the pathologist measures the biopsy and puts ink on the surface

ink

normal breast tissue

tumor

lumpectomy specimen

lumpectomy is sliced into sections

tumor present at inked margin

each slice is examined by the pathologist grossly and under a microscope to determine if the tumor extends to the margin when you consider the difference between DCIS and invasive cancer; in invasive cancer, the cancers cells go through all the breast tissue, instead of being contained within the duct system and normal areas of breast tissue are interspersed between ducts containing DCIS.

CAROL IS FIFTY-SIX, and a very busy corporate attorney. It's not uncommon for her to be on and off her cell phone during our appointments. She was raised in Alabama and has a wonderful accent. When I met her for her first visit she was very formal and reserved, firmly declaring, "Dr. Chan, I *am* an attorney but I do *not* participate in malpractice law." It's sadly humorous that often my attorney patients feel that they have to say something like that. I'm certainly not going to give them anything less than my best, regardless.

Today I'm seeing Carol for her postoperative check. Several weeks ago, she had a lumpectomy with sentinel lymph node biopsy. She's a large imposing woman wearing business attire and holding a bulging briefcase on her lap. Of course, she is on her phone.

After saying hello, I tell her that I'll step out while she puts on a gown so that I can examine her. While still holding the phone and ignoring the person on the other end of her call, she stops in mid-sentence to keep me from leaving, and loudly exclaims in her Southern accent, "Lordy, what in heaven for? This month, I've had nearly a hundred people peak at my boobs! Here, let me just lift up my blouse." She suddenly remembers her phone call and speaks into the phone, "Oh, I'm at my doctor's appointment." She then lifts up her blouse and bra with her free hand and says to me, "You were absolutely, positively right. That surgeon did one hell of a job."

Carol's operated breast matches her other breast very well. She has a small incision like a thin crescent moon just above her areola that is still blue from the sentinel node injection. The blue will fade over a couple of months. She has another small incision healing under her armpit.

Her pathology report indicates that the margins are clear and that the sentinel nodes are negative. When she ends her call, I review the results with her (we are both pleased) and tell her that her surgery is complete and that we can move on with her other treatments.

Q *What is wire localization lumpectomy or excision?*

A Often, a breast cancer cannot be felt by the surgeon and is detectable only by mammogram or ultrasound. In order to locate the cancer for removal by lumpectomy, one or two wires are placed into the breast near the cancer by the radiologist to provide the surgeon with a target for the lumpectomy. The removed specimen is typically X-rayed to confirm that the cancer is within the specimen. In situations where the surgeon can detect the cancer by touch, this technique is not needed.

Q *What is a mastectomy?*

A This is complete surgical removal of the breast and is required when the size of the cancer compared to the size of the breast is too large to permit a lumpectomy. A successful lumpectomy requires both safety (from the standpoint of having clear margins), and also a good cosmetic appearance. If this cannot be achieved, mastectomy is required.

Mastectomy is also required in situations where there is more than one cancer within the breast, particularly if the cancers occur in different sections or quadrants. This is called multicentric breast cancer and the standard of care is mastectomy. When there are two separate cancers within the same area of the breast, it's called multifocal. Some multifocal cancers can be treated successfully with lumpectomy and radiation if the cancers are close together and a reasonably sized lumpectomy can completely remove them with clear margins.

Mastectomy is accomplished by removing the entire breast tissue, which includes the skin, the fat, and areola with the nipple. The chest muscles aren't removed so there shouldn't be functional weakness of the arm or shoulder. The final surgical result is the complete absence of the breast, with a horizontal scar across the underlying chest area.

MONICA IS FORTY-FIVE, the mother of three young children. I'm seeing her today for her four-year checkup. When she was forty-one, she had the misfortune of having bilateral breast cancers. Her right breast cancer was large, 6 cm, and her left breast cancer was much smaller, 1 cm. Her breast size was relatively small.

During the initial consultations, I had discussed with Monica and Jim, her husband, the possibility of using preoperative chemotherapy to try to avoid mastectomy on the larger cancer on the right. I explained, however, that because the right cancer was large compared to her breast size, there was a high chance that despite preoperative chemotherapy, she'd still need a mastectomy. In the left breast with the small cancer, she could have had a lumpectomy and radiation for breast conservation.

Following a lengthy discussion on the surgery options, Monica tentatively indicated that she was considering mastectomy on both sides. She would then delay a tissue reconstruction so that she could minimize the amount of surgery needed and still care for her children. I still remember how she looked at her husband as she said this, trying to sense his reaction. Jim, a big man, turned to her and said softly, "Hey Moni, it doesn't really matter to me. You know it's not going to change how I feel about you. All I want is for you to be well. That is the only thing that's important."

On today's visit, four years later, Monica hasn't yet had reconstruction. I ask her if she is still considering it. She replies, "You know, when I decided to have the mastectomies, I was sure that I was going to do it, the reconstruction thing. With time, I thought about it less and less. Now I'm happy just the way I am and Jim never says anything about it. I guess I'm just too busy with the kids and all and don't have time for the surgeries. I still might do it later."

Q *What is an axillary lymph node dissection?*
A An axillary node dissection involves removal of a specific area of fat under the armpit. This area is connected to the upper outer portion of the breast and contains the lymph nodes into which breast cancer can initially spread. Everyone will have a different number of nodes within the axillary dissection specimen and an axillary node dissection should not remove all the lymph nodes under the armpit. On average the number of nodes can be between eight and twenty-five. The surgeon does not know how many nodes have been removed by the operation until the pathologist examines the specimen.

Unfortunately as a result of this surgery, there is permanent

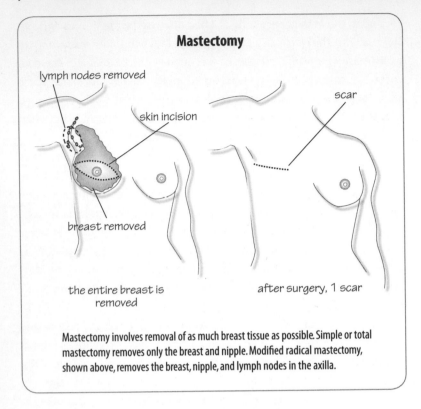

Mastectomy

lymph nodes removed

skin incision

scar

breast removed

the entire breast is
removed

after surgery, 1 scar

Mastectomy involves removal of as much breast tissue as possible. Simple or total
mastectomy removes only the breast and nipple. Modified radical mastectomy,
shown above, removes the breast, nipple, and lymph nodes in the axilla.

numbness in the armpit and temporary numbness in the inner upper
arm. Over time, some patients can develop significant swelling of
the arm and hand, a process called lymphedema. Fortunately, severe
lymphedema is uncommon. See chapter 17 for a discussion of lymphedema prevention. Another possible side effect is long-term pain
across the chest, related to cutting of nerves that normally go across
the chest from the armpit. When this type of pain occurs, it usually
begins several months after surgery, not right away.

When an axillary lymph node dissection is performed with a
lumpectomy, the best cosmetic results occur when the surgeon
makes two separate incisions rather than trying to encompass both
the lumpectomy and node dissection within one incision. Two
separate smaller incisions generally result in less scarring within

the breast with radiation therapy compared to one large incision and results in the breast having a better appearance after radiation therapy.

For invasive breast cancers, it's important to know whether or not the cancer has spread to the draining lymph nodes within the armpit (the axilla) to permit accurate planning of therapy. Axillary node dissection usually isn't performed for DCIS because it isn't invasive and therefore shouldn't spread.

Q *What is a sentinel node biopsy?*
A This is a relatively new technique for determining whether invasive breast cancer has spread into the lymph nodes within the armpit and again usually involves a second incision under the armpit. The procedure is usually performed at the same time as a lumpectomy or mastectomy and was designed to limit the discomfort and lymphedema risk associated with an axillary node dissection. The technique was actually developed by surgeons operating on a type of aggressive skin cancer called melanoma.

The goal is to locate the initial draining lymph nodes of the breast within the armpit and to remove them without cutting nerves and affecting the normal lymph node drainage of the arm. A blue dye and a radioactive tracer are injected into the breast. There are two ways to perform the injection, either around the location of the cancer or around the areola. Both ways seem to be equally effective. While an instrument is used to find the radioactive tracer within the armpit, a small incision is made and only the blue nodes stained by blue dye are removed. These blue nodes are the sentinel nodes, and represent the first draining nodes from the cancer and from the breast. The sentinel nodes can't always be found, but an experienced surgeon should be able to find them 95 percent of the time. Several studies now show that the test is very accurate in assessing whether or not there is spread into lymph nodes. With only a sentinel node biopsy, the chance of long-term pain or lymphedema is much less than with an axillary node dissection and occurs very rarely.

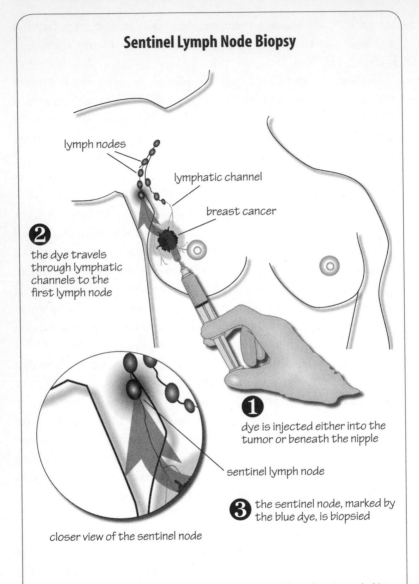

Sentinel Lymph Node Biopsy

lymph nodes

lymphatic channel

breast cancer

2 the dye travels through lymphatic channels to the first lymph node

1 dye is injected either into the tumor or beneath the nipple

sentinel lymph node

3 the sentinel node, marked by the blue dye, is biopsied

closer view of the sentinel node

Sentinel lymph node biopsy involves injecting dye (sometimes with a radioactive marker) into either the tumor or beneath the nipple. The dye drains from the breast into lymphatic vessels which carry the dye to the first lymph node, called the sentinel node. This node is then biopsied. The pathologist examines the sentinel node for metastatic carcinoma.

Q *Do patients who undergo sentinel node biopsy ever need to have an axillary lymph node dissection?*

A There are several reasons why an axillary dissection may be needed. During sentinel node surgery, the sentinel nodes are examined by the pathologist using a preliminary evaluation called a frozen section. If cancer is detected in the sentinel nodes, an axillary lymph node dissection is performed right then. Often the frozen section analysis shows no cancer, but later analysis with special staining or molecular techniques does reveal cancer. When this happens, a discussion takes place with the patient about whether or not a second operation is required to do an axillary lymph node dissection.

This question is currently being studied in a national clinical trial conducted by the American College of Surgeons, and is a controversial question about which experts have heated discussions. If the amount of cancer within the sentinel node is very small, I usually do not recommend an axillary node dissection because I am in the group of experts who feel that an axillary node dissection is a test for cancer spread, rather than a treatment that will improve cure rate. Other experts may disagree and feel that the axillary lymph node dissection is of therapeutic value, that having an axillary dissection will improve cure rates. However, most studies do not support the viewpoint that the surgery has therapeutic value because improved survival rates are not demonstrated in clinical trials of axillary dissection. When compared to the groups of patients who haven't undergone axillary dissection, the survivals are the same. Therefore if axillary dissection has therapeutic value, the benefit is probably fairly small.

Q *What is mastectomy with immediate reconstruction?*

A Patients who undergo mastectomy are often given the option of immediate (simultaneous) reconstruction with a plastic surgeon. This usually results in better breast contour and shape compared with delayed reconstruction because more normal skin can be left by the surgeon, a so-called skin-sparing mastectomy. This requires a skilled plastic surgeon who can perform the reconstruction with either a breast implant or with the patient's own tissue removed from another

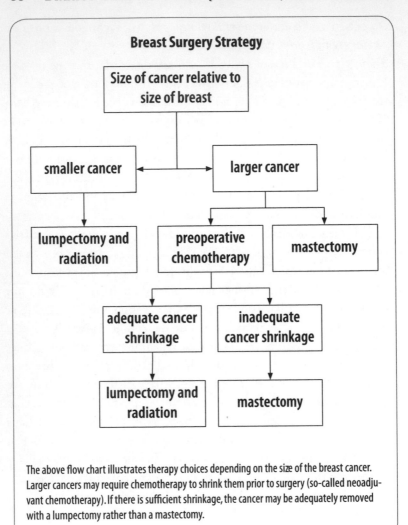

Breast Surgery Strategy

The above flow chart illustrates therapy choices depending on the size of the breast cancer. Larger cancers may require chemotherapy to shrink them prior to surgery (so-called neoadjuvant chemotherapy). If there is sufficient shrinkage, the cancer may be adequately removed with a lumpectomy rather than a mastectomy.

area, usually the fat from the lower abdominal area. Studies show that there is no more breast tissue left behind in a skin-sparing mastectomy with immediate reconstruction compared to a standard mastectomy. Therefore, skin-sparing mastectomy with immediate reconstruction is considered as safe as a mastectomy with delayed reconstruction, but has the benefit of having a better cosmetic result.

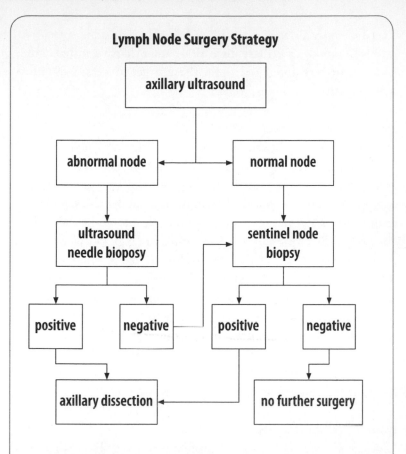

Lymph Node Surgery Strategy

The above flow chart illustrates therapy choices based on the finding of an abnormal lymph node in the axilla (arm pit). The lymph node may be found by physician examination or may be visible using ultrasound. The lymph node is biopsied and depending on whether or not metastatic cancer is found in the lymph node, more surgery may be required to removed many of the lymph nodes in the axilla (so called axillary dissection).

Q *What is a modified radical mastectomy?*

A This is a mastectomy, complete removal of the breast, combined with an axillary lymph node dissection. This surgery is needed when a patient has a large cancer compared to breast size and when there is known lymph node involvement prior to surgery. Sometimes the lymph nodes are found to be abnormal by mammogram or ultrasound and a needle biopsy, prior to surgery, confirms that spread has occurred. In this situation, an axillary dissection rather than a sentinel lymph node biopsy is required and so for these larger cancers, a modified radical mastectomy is performed.

Q *What is a radical mastectomy?*

A This was a type of mastectomy performed in the 1950s and 1960s, and involved a mastectomy with a complete lymph node dissection as well as removal of the underlying chest muscle. The surgeon would attempt to remove every single lymph node under the armpit and would also remove the entire chest muscle, the pectoralis major. This was a very debilitating surgery that resulted in a high rate of long-term pain, arm weakness, and also arm swelling (lymphedema). A radical mastectomy is no longer performed because studies have shown no advantage over a modified radical mastectomy which leaves the chest muscles intact and removes fewer lymph nodes. When mastectomy and node removal are needed, the current surgery is a modified radical mastectomy. Modified radical mastectomy is just as effective in treating breast cancer, and the more limited surgery results in much less pain and a much lower chance of arm swelling.

Q *What can I do to help prepare for surgery?*

A Unless you have other medical problems, it's very likely that your surgery will be done as an outpatient. This means that you will check into the hospital or surgical center several hours prior to the operation. You will be instructed to not eat or drink anything after midnight on the evening prior to surgery. If you need to take medication in the morning of surgery, ask your surgeon whether the medication should be skipped, or whether you should take the medication with a small amount of water.

After the operation, you will be in the recovery area for several hours until the effects of anesthesia wear off. You will need transportation home, because you will not be permitted to drive yourself due to possible lingering effects of the anesthesia. If you are having a lumpectomy, you should purchase two cotton sport bras (without underwire) that fasten in the front. This will provide helpful support

after surgery. You need a bra that fastens in the front if y
a sentinel node biopsy or an axillary dissection because
initially unable to reach around to your back because of the
under your armpit. There's a good chance you will be sent home with
a drain or two in place. These are temporary soft plastic tubes that
help to reduce swelling. Make sure that you have clear instructions
on how to take care of the drains. It's not complicated, but you do
need to be told what to do, how to empty the drains, and how to
keep the area clean.

Q *After breast surgery, do I need to have radiation therapy?*

A If you have a lumpectomy, breast radiation is almost always given to
reduce the risk of cancer coming back within the breast. Of course
there are exceptions to this, such as a small low grade DCIS that
has been removed with widely clear margins. Also, recent studies
indicate that older patients with small invasive cancers removed by
lumpectomy may be given the option of omitting radiation. This is
somewhat controversial and requires significant discussion before
making a decision to forego radiation if you have had a lumpectomy
for an invasive breast cancer.

If you have a mastectomy, radiation is usually given under two
circumstances; if the cancer is 5 cm or larger or if more than 3 lymph
nodes contain cancer. Radiation therapy after mastectomy for these
situations has been shown to reduce the recurrences within the mastectomy scar and also seem to reduce the spread of breast cancer.

8

※

What Are My Choices for Reconstruction after Mastectomy?

Q *What are the reasons for needing to have a mastectomy?*

A The main reason for mastectomy is the need to completely remove the breast because the cancer, compared to breast size, is too large to allow for a lumpectomy with an acceptable cosmetic result. Or in other words, the lumpectomy required to remove a big cancer removes too much of the breast, causing significant deformity of the breast shape.

A second common reason for needing a mastectomy is when a lumpectomy is unsuccessful in clearing margins. Although re-excision, an attempt to complete the lumpectomy, can be tried once or twice more, eventually the remaining breast becomes cosmetically unacceptable and a mastectomy is required.

There are also patients who choose to have a mastectomy instead of breast conservation. For some women, this choice is made from fear of having a breast that once had cancer in it. For some, this fear still remains despite numerous studies demonstrating equal safety for breast conservation compared to mastectomy. For these women, a mastectomy is a more emotionally comfortable option. Other women may not want to have radiation therapy and therefore also choose to have a mastectomy.

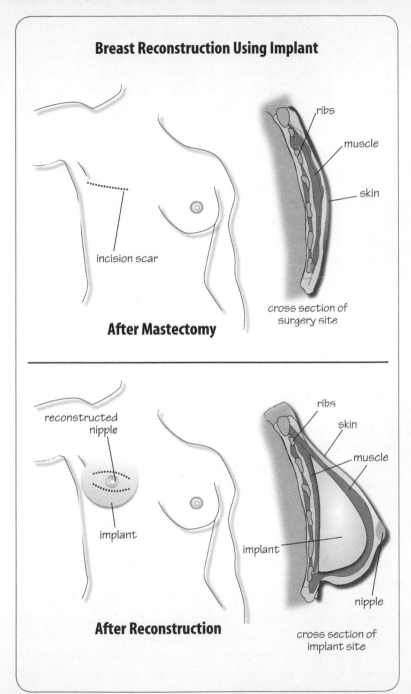

Breast Reconstruction Using Implant

ribs

muscle

skin

incision scar

cross section of
surgery site

After Mastectomy

reconstructed
nipple

ribs

skin

muscle

implant

implant

nipple

After Reconstruction

cross section of
implant site

Q *If I need a mastectomy, should I have immediate reconstruction?*

A Immediate reconstruction refers to having reconstruction of the breast performed immediately, during the surgery for mastectomy rather than later with a second operation. If it's likely that you won't need radiation therapy after mastectomy, immediate reconstruction should be considered because the cosmetic result is usually better. This is because the plastic surgeon is able to use more of the normal skin of the breast. If you need radiation after mastectomy because the cancer is greater than 5 cm or more than 3 nodes are involved, reconstruction should probably be delayed because radiation may affect the appearance and feel of the reconstructed breast.

If you choose immediate reconstruction, the primary surgeon will perform a mastectomy with either a sentinel node biopsy or an axillary dissection. During the same surgery, the plastic surgeon then reconstructs the breast immediately following mastectomy. The advantage to this approach is a better cosmetic result because the skin on the lower part of the mastectomy area is saved, permitting a more natural drop and more realistic shape for the reconstructed breast. This is called a skin-sparing mastectomy with immediate reconstruction, and usually results in a more natural appearing reconstructed breast.

Q *What type of reconstruction should I have? Should I consider reconstruction with an implant?*

A Breast reconstruction is performed with either an implant or with your own tissue moved from another area of your body. As you probably know, an implant is basically a plastic bag filled either with silicone, which is a liquid plastic, or saline, which is salt water. The advantage of an implant over tissue reconstruction is that the surgery is simpler, quicker, and the healing time is faster. Silicone implants tend to have a feel that is more like normal breast tissue in comparison to saline implants. Silicone implants are FDA approved for breast reconstruction following mastectomy. They are not approved for routine breast enlargement. Although there has been frequently publicized concern in the lay media about the safety of silicone implants, multiple studies in the U.S. and Europe now consistently demonstrate a very high level of safety for this device.

Implant reconstruction involves first placing what is called a tissue expander underneath the mastectomy incision. The tissue expander is a flat plastic balloon that contains a valve through which the balloon is gradually inflated with saline over several months. This stretches the skin and allows comfortable placement of the implant. When adequate expansion is achieved, a second surgery is performed to remove the tissue expander and replace it with the breast implant. A subsequent third operation is performed to reconstruct the nipple area by pulling up a section of skin. Tattooing around the reconstructed nipple recreates the areola. A realistic reconstruction requires multiple surgeries.

Many implant reconstructions are cosmetically successful. The disadvantage of implants is that they are fairly firm compared to normal breast tissue and this becomes noticeable if people hug you. Also as you move, the implant tends not to move as a normal breast would. There is also sometimes a need for re-operation due to either implant leakage or the development of a capsular contracture. Capsular contracture refers to a buildup of scar tissue around the implant that makes it uncomfortable and very firm. The rate of re-operation may be as high as 50 percent over a ten-year period, although the surgery is relatively easy and brief.

Q *Why should I avoid implant reconstruction if I need radiation therapy after mastectomy?*

A Some patients have large cancers or many involved lymph nodes. As I have discussed before, the current standard is that after a mastectomy, if the cancer is 5 cm or greater, or if there are more than 3 involved lymph nodes, then radiation therapy is needed to reduce the chance of cancer recurrence. The radiation is given over six weeks to the skin of the mastectomy scar, under part of the armpit where the lymph nodes reside (the axilla), and above the collar bone (the supraclavicular area) where there is also lymph node drainage from the breast. The radiation causes the skin to become stiffer and non-pliable and an implant in this situation tends to be very uncomfortable and very firm. Patients who undergo reconstruction and are likely to need radiation afterward should have a delayed reconstruction. When radiation is needed after mastectomy, the majority of plastic surgeons prefer to use a patient's own tissue, so-called autologous tissue reconstruction rather than an implant.

Q *What is a TRAM reconstruction?*

A This is the most common type of autologous tissue reconstruction using abdominal tissue, the area over your belly. TRAM stands for transverse rectus abdominis musculocutaneous and refers to the area from where the tissue is removed, namely the skin of part of the lower abdomen with underlying fat and part of the rectus (abdominal) muscle. This can be performed as an immediate reconstruction or as a delayed reconstruction following radiation.

The surgery does require a different type of skill compared to implant reconstruction and is conceptually rather amazing. Fat, skin, and muscle with the blood vessels attached are separated from the front of the abdomen in what is called a pedicle or flap. This is tunneled underneath the upper abdomen and positioned in the mastectomy scar. Most of the breast is reconstructed with abdominal fat so that the patient also has what is essentially a "tummy tuck." The abdominal incision is similar in location to that of a C-section. TRAM reconstructive surgery may take five to six hours. The healing of the abdominal incision from where the tissue was removed may take four to six weeks. Again, later the nipple and areola are reconstructed surgically by pulling up extra skin and tattooing the area around it. The contour of the reconstructed breast is often excellent and has the advantage of feeling like normal breast tissue. It is soft to the touch and will move like a normal breast under clothing. There was initially some concern that splitting the abdominal muscle would lead to abdominal weakness, but that doesn't seem to be a significant problem for most patients, even those who are athletic.

A newer variation of this technique is a DIEP (deep inferior epigastric perforator) flap, which basically uses only abdominal skin and fat without muscle. The name refers to the blood vessel from the front of the abdomen that is used to nourish the flap. This technique is also called a free flap, because it is completely unattached when it is moved and the blood vessels are completely severed. The free flap graft of

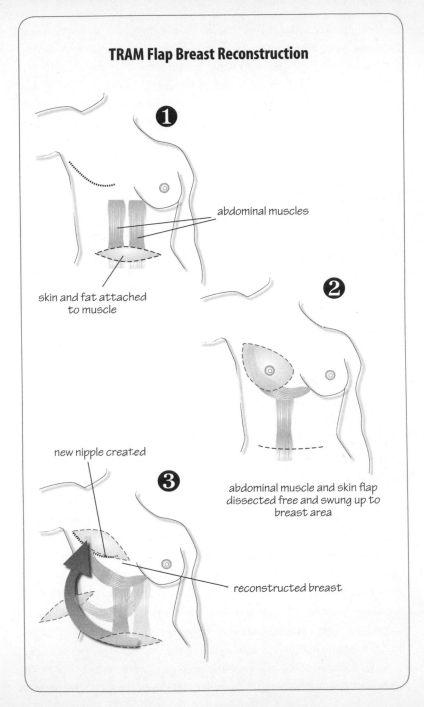

TRAM Flap Breast Reconstruction

❶

abdominal muscles

skin and fat attached
to muscle

❷

abdominal muscle and skin flap
dissected free and swung up to
breast area

new nipple created

❸

reconstructed breast

abdominal skin and fat is reattached using microsurgical technique to reattach the blood vessels of the flap to those on the chest wall. The plastic surgeon uses an operating microscope to meticulously reattach the flap to small blood vessels of the chest. Compared to TRAM reconstruction, DIEP flap reconstruction requires an extra level of expertise and technique on the part of the plastic surgeon and not all plastic surgeons are trained to perform this.

※

LOUISE IS SIXTY-THREE years old. I had treated her three years ago for a large cancer of the right breast that required a mastectomy, six months of chemotherapy, and radiation to the mastectomy incision. She is single, has two adult children, and works as an analyst for a defense contractor. As in previous visits, she has come from work dressed in business attire and I ask her to change into a gown for examination.

What seems different with Louise on her visit today is that she's very bubbly. Several months ago she underwent a TRAM reconstruction of her right breast and she's eager to show me the results. Louise is five feet eight inches tall and about 135 pounds. She removes her gown and stands very straight. Where before she had a mastectomy scar across her right chest, she now has a natural appearing breast contour that is actually somewhat larger than her left breast.

"Dr. White said he'll liposuction it to make it smaller in a couple of months so that it'll match better. I asked him if he could inject the extra fat into the left one," she says with a small laugh.

I ask Louise if she's happy with the early results. "Absolutely! But what's most amazing to me is my belly where the fat came from. I can't believe how flat it is. Look at it! It's not been like that since I was twenty."

Louise is pleased and absolutely beaming. I ask her if she wouldn't mind showing her surgery results to Connie, a patient in an adjacent exam room. It has become apparent to me that Connie is going to need a mastectomy because we couldn't clear margins after an initial lumpectomy and a second large re-excision. Louise agrees to show her reconstruction to Connie and puts the gown back on, open in front.

As we step out of the exam room to walk to Connie's room, we pass by one of my senior partners, Dr. Greening. He gives me a puzzled look as he sees me with a patient in a gown walking down the halls of the cancer center. As we pass by, I tell him we are going to see another patient to show her Louise's reconstruction. Before he can reply, Louise spins around toward him and throws open her gown like a flasher while saying, "What do you think?"

Dr. Greening is startled and taken aback. After a moment or two, he blushes, looks down quickly at his shoes, and mumbles, "Very nice."

Q *What if I am too thin for a TRAM or DIEP flap reconstruction?*

A There are other options for autologous tissue reconstruction if you are too thin to donate enough abdominal fat to re-create a breast mound. One technique is to transfer tissue from underneath the back part of the shoulder, a latissimus myocutaneous flap which uses part of the latissimus dorsi muscle. This is the muscle that makes up the back part of your armpit. Sometimes even tissue from the buttocks is used, which is called a gluteal flap. Again the advantage of this type of reconstruction is that the reconstructed breast feels like normal tissue and the reconstruction can be performed even when radiation is needed. Some very thin women require a latissimus flap with the addition of a small implant as well.

Q *My physicians tell me that I'll need radiation after mastectomy but I want immediate reconstruction. What are the potential problems?*

A As a general rule, the reconstruction should be with your own tissue and not an implant as mentioned above because of the likelihood of fibrosis and scarring resulting from radiation. An implant in this situation is usually too firm and uncomfortable. There is some experience with giving radiation to patients who have had immediate reconstruction with TRAM and DIEP flaps. The cosmetic results can be good but there is a higher chance of developing areas of hardness within the reconstructed breast. Also, modifications of the flap after radiation are generally more difficult and tend to heal very slowly.

However, there is a new technique being introduced called delayed-immediate breast reconstruction, a rather unusual name. This was recently described by Dr. Steven Kronowitz from M. D. Anderson

Cancer Center in Houston. During mastectomy, a skin sparing procedure is performed using a tissue expander. The skin of the breast and the expander underneath is then radiated. After the radiation effects have subsided, the expander is removed and the final tissue reconstruction is performed. This seems to give an overall better cosmetic result. It's a very new technique and seems to make sense but more studies will be needed before it becomes widely accepted.

Q *How do I select a plastic surgeon?*

A A good place to start is to ask your surgeon who he or she would recommend and schedule a consultation appointment. A good plastic surgeon will show you photos of other patients who have had the type of reconstruction you are considering, and may also tell you why you shouldn't have a certain type of reconstruction. Optimally, you would have the chance to meet some other patients so that you can see and even feel the final result. I think that is very helpful and you should ask if this is possible.

It's important to understand that not every plastic surgeon is expert in every type of reconstruction and it's probably better for you to change plastic surgeons or obtain second opinions rather than insist on a type of reconstruction that your surgeon isn't enthusiastic about. It's very disheartening to go through a lot of surgery and end up with a poor reconstruction.

9

✳

What Is Meant by Staging and Why Is It Important?

Q *What is meant by staging?*

A Staging is the process of estimating the extent of a cancer in order to assess relapse risk and to permit proper treatment planning. The staging system for different cancer types is specific for that cancer because different factors are important in predicting survival. Higher stages of a cancer are usually associated with a lower chance of survival. Therefore the staging of breast cancer is unique to breast cancer and can be used to predict the possibilities for cure. This allows treatments to be planned accordingly.

Q *How is breast cancer staged?*

A The TNM staging system is used to separate the stages into four groups, often denoted by Roman numerals. The T stage denotes the size of the cancer within the breast, the N stage whether or not lymph nodes are involved, and the M stage indicates whether the cancer has spread beyond the breast and lymph nodes. Stages I, II, and III indicate higher TNM stages with increasing amounts of cancer within the breast and nodes. In the TNM system, if the M has the number 1 next to it, it signifies stage IV disease, denoting widespread or metastatic breast cancer. Therefore No indicates that no lymph nodes are involved and Mo indicates that there is not detectable spread to other areas of the body.

Q *Why is staging important?*

A The stage determines the level of danger the cancer poses and influences the treatment strategy needed for optimal outcomes. Lower stage breast cancers have better cure rates and require less treatment to achieve cure. Having stage IV disease is very unfortunate because with currently available treatments, metastatic breast cancer is not considered potentially curable and a different treatment approach is needed. Having said that, it is important to emphasize that patients with metastatic breast cancer can survive many years and have very good quality of life with treatments now available.

Disease stages I, II, and III can be cured with existing therapies, but achieving cure requires more intensive treatment with higher stages. Basically, the stage helps us determine how curable the cancer is and how much treatment is needed for cure.

Q *How is stage established?*

A Stages I, II, and III are determined by the pathologist after primary breast surgery, which can be either a lumpectomy or a mastectomy and some type of surgical lymph node analysis. This is really where the importance of either a sentinel node biopsy or axillary dissection comes into play in invasive breast cancer. Although the size of the breast cancer can be estimated using mammogram or ultrasound, it is only accurately determined under the microscope because some cancers have small fingerlike extensions that are too fine to be seen by an X-ray or scan. Similarly, although mammogram and ultrasound may indicate normal lymph nodes, very small amounts of cancer within the nodes can be detected by the pathologist using special staining techniques and a microscope. Mammograms and ultrasounds are unable to see the minute amounts of cancer visible only under the microscope. Therefore, although stage can be roughly estimated before surgery, it is only definitively determined following complete analysis of the surgical specimen by the pathologist.

Q *How are patients diagnosed with stage IV disease?*

A This is somewhat more problematic. Stage IV denotes metastatic disease, which means that breast cancer has spread beyond the breast and immediate draining lymph nodes. The way the cancer spreads is through the lymphatic system or blood stream to other organs. Metastatic breast cancer is typically detected by a scan. However some abnormal scans are equivocal or may be abnormal for reasons other than cancer. When abnormal scans are less than definitive, a biopsy can be confirmatory.

Q *Should I be getting routine body and bone scans now that I've been diagnosed with breast cancer?*

A According to the current national guidelines, if you are the average breast cancer patient, you should not get routine scans. There are a number of good reasons for not scanning every patient routinely. It's very rare for a newly diagnosed breast cancer patient with early stage disease (stage I or II) to have metastatic breast cancer detectable by currently available scanning technology. If spread of cancer has occurred in early stage breast cancer, it is by and large microscopic and too small for a scan to pick up.

The majority of patients with metastatic breast cancer are patients who have relapsed a number of years following initial treatment for early stage disease. Newly diagnosed breast cancer with metastatic stage IV disease is fortunately fairly uncommon.

The problem with the currently available scans is that they have significant inaccuracies. Every medical test or scan can have abnormalities due to non-cancerous reasons (false positive), and alternatively, can be inaccurately normal because the amount of cancer present is below the detectable range of the scan (false negative). This creates a dilemma because an inaccurate scan result could lead to improper treatment decisions. In addition to resulting in patients receiving unnecessary radiation, overuse of scanning tests sometimes can result in incorrect treatment decisions as a consequence of the inaccuracies of the tests.

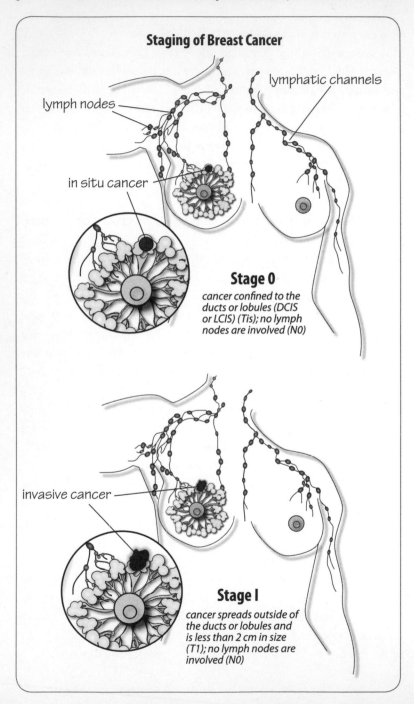

Staging of Breast Cancer

lymph nodes

lymphatic channels

in situ cancer

Stage 0
cancer confined to the ducts or lobules (DCIS or LCIS) (Tis); no lymph nodes are involved (N0)

invasive cancer

Stage I
cancer spreads outside of the ducts or lobules and is less than 2 cm in size (T1); no lymph nodes are involved (N0)

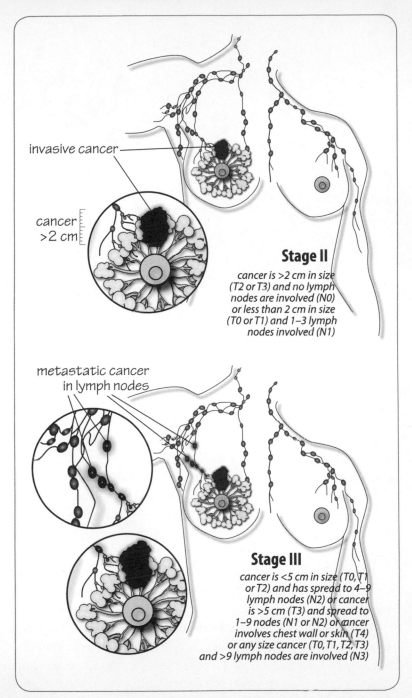

invasive cancer

cancer
>2 cm

Stage II

*cancer is >2 cm in size
(T2 or T3) and no lymph
nodes are involved (N0)
or less than 2 cm in size
(T0 or T1) and 1–3 lymph
nodes involved (N1)*

metastatic cancer
in lymph nodes

Stage III

*cancer is <5 cm in size (T0, T1
or T2) and has spread to 4–9
lymph nodes (N2) or cancer
is >5 cm (T3) and spread to
1–9 nodes (N1 or N2) or cancer
involves chest wall or skin (T4)
or any size cancer (T0, T1, T2, T3)
and >9 lymph nodes are involved (N3)*

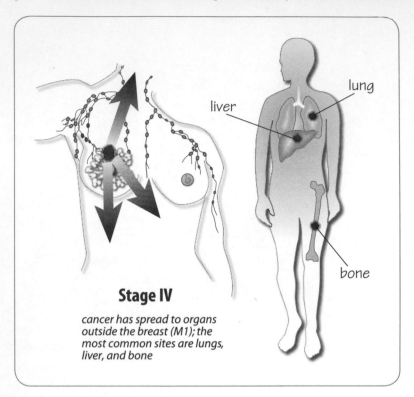

liver

lung

bone

Stage IV

cancer has spread to organs outside the breast (M1); the most common sites are lungs, liver, and bone

Q *What are the scans most used in breast cancer?*

A A CT (CAT scan) uses X-rays to create a computer-based image as you lie down and go through a large X-ray tube. The MRI is a computer-generated scan created by changes in electromagnetic fields rather than X-rays as you go through a tube containing a powerful magnet. A PET scan uses differences in sugar (glucose) uptake between cancer cells and normal cells to create a computerized image in a process similar to undergoing a CT scan.

A bone scan is a test using an injection of radioactive material that is taken up by bone areas that are metabolically active and can be seen with a special camera.

All of these tests are limited by the inability to reliably detect cancer smaller than one cubic centimeter, roughly the diameter of your little fingernail. One cubic centimeter of cancer represents a tumor volume of one billion cancer cells, which is quite a significant amount of cancer to miss. Therefore a patient could have many nodules of metastatic cancer that are 2 to 3 mm in size and have completely normal CT, MRI, PET, and bone scans. There are many false negative tests.

Equally important, none of these scans are specific for breast cancer, or for that matter any other type of cancer, and can be abnormal for benign (non-cancerous) reasons. There are significant numbers of false positive tests. For example, abnormalities on CT or MRI can be due to normal variations in anatomy such as benign cysts. PET scans can be abnormal due to infections or areas of inflammation. Bone scans are often abnormal because of areas of arthritis or bone injury. So these scans are inaccurate and can either underestimate or overestimate breast cancer stage. This is why they aren't currently recommended for the average early stage newly diagnosed breast cancer patient or for regular use during routine follow-up.

LIZA IS PRESENT with her adult daughter, Mara. They're both very blond, slightly heavy, and appear more like sisters. Liza recently had a small left breast cancer removed by lumpectomy and had sentinel node biopsy. On her current chest X-ray, she is found to have a small abnormality in her right lung. A subsequent CT scan reveals several additional nodules, each about a centimeter in size, in both lungs.

Prior to their visit, Liza and Mara have obtained the radiologist's report, which reads "consistent with metastatic disease" because this pattern is typical for a spreading cancer. She and her daughter are understandably quite upset. I usually don't like patients having their own reports prior to discussing the results with a physician, because a scan report needs to be put into proper context. I explain to them that although the scan result is worrisome, it's possible that the abnormalities result from something other than metastatic breast cancer because Liza's breast cancer is small and her sentinel nodes are normal. She has what should be an early stage breast cancer.

I order a PET scan, which unfortunately is also abnormal in both lungs. Again the report by the radiologist states, "consistent with metastatic cancer." Liza and Mara want her to begin chemotherapy immediately. I caution them that the abnormal PET scan has me more worried, but I still believe there's a possibility of causes other than cancer. Because her situation is atypical for what should have been a favorable breast cancer, I recommend a CT guided needle biopsy and Liza agrees.

As the radiologist sets Liza up for the CT biopsy, he notes that although the spots are still there, they seem to be getting smaller and calls me to ask if he should proceed. I discuss the scan improvements with Liza by phone but we decide to go ahead with the biopsy because she can't deal with the uncertainty of not knowing what is going on. When Liza and her daughter return to see me three days later, I inform them that the biopsy shows a fungal infection and no cancer. We're all very relieved. Rather than receiving chemotherapy for metastatic breast cancer, I arrange for her to see an infectious disease specialist and she takes post-lumpectomy radiation and Arimidex. A follow-up CT scan six months later is normal.

The important lesson here is that radiology tests are not specifically cancer tests. They are tests that show anatomic or functional abnormalities and require thoughtful interpretation by the treating physician. Be careful not to jump to conclusions.

Q *Which newly diagnosed patients should be considered for these types of scans?*

A CT scans are typically reserved for patients who have locally advanced breast cancer, stage III. These are patients with cancer larger than 5 cm, or more than 3 involved lymph nodes, or a less common condition called inflammatory breast cancer. Again, any abnormality on scan may represent a non-cancer situation so that if technically possible, biopsy to confirm metastatic disease should be considered if the results are unclear. It's currently not established whether patients with stage III breast cancer should have PET scans. It's possible that PET scans may detect earlier metastatic breast cancer compared to CT scans. Whether this would be advantageous to know is unclear and for the moment PET scans in newly diagnosed stage III patients with normal CT scans aren't routinely performed. We don't yet know whether patients who are stage IV by only PET scan, all other tests being normal, are incurable or not because information on cure rates and stage so far have only been reported with the use of CT and not PET scans.

Q *What about blood tests or tumor markers? What are they and how are they used?*

A It would be very helpful to have a blood test that could diagnose cancer or help stage your cancer. A tumor marker refers to a blood test that measures any protein produced by cancer cells that is released into the blood stream. The markers most studied for breast cancer are CEA, CA15–3, and CA 27–29. Many studies unfortunately show that these markers are inaccurate in measuring breast cancer. Patients can have normal markers in the setting of metastatic disease (false negative), and elevations of markers for benign reasons (false positive). For example, a previous history of smoking can cause long-term elevation of CEA. All of the national cancer organizations and study groups currently recommend against routine monitoring of blood tumor markers for breast cancer because they have been unreliable and have generally not helped find metastatic cancer that would not have been found by other means.

Q *How does a bone scan differ from a bone density test?*

A A bone scan is a nuclear medicine test using a short-lived mildly radio-active substance injected intravenously. Two hours later, photos are taken with a special camera revealing areas of abnormal bone activity. The areas of abnormal bone activity may be from any cause, not only cancer, including areas of arthritis, trauma from previous injuries or fractures, and also areas of cancer involving the bones. Studies revealing the inaccuracy of bone scans show that if you have no new or increasing bone pain, any area of abnormality on bone scan has a better than 90 percent chance of being due to arthritis or old injury rather than metastatic breast cancer. There is a very high false positive rate, meaning that in the majority of cases the abnormality on the test isn't due to cancer. A bone density X-ray is not a cancer test at all and isn't used for cancer detection. It measures the thickness of your bones and assesses whether or not you have osteoporosis, a condition of bone softening.

Q *What about bone marrow analysis?*

A At present this is a research tool in breast cancer. The bone marrow is the center part of the bone where blood is made and can be tested by removing a sample from the back of the pelvic bone using a biopsy needle. With the use of special staining technique, tests in breast cancer patients show that some newly diagnosed breast cancer patients have small amounts of breast cancer in the bone marrow. Relatively long-term follow-up of these patients, however, shows that the majority of patients with microscopic breast cancer metastasis in the bone marrow don't relapse and have a relapse rate only slightly higher than those with normal marrows. This is a somewhat unexpected finding and hard to explain. Therefore, at present, the significance of minimal bone marrow involvement by individual breast cancer cells is uncertain. It may be that at a later date with more studies, this test may be useful in determining which patients who are lymph node negative require chemotherapy. For now, bone marrow assessment is not being performed outside of a clinical trial.

Q *So for the average newly diagnosed breast cancer patient, the staging is primarily determined by the results of the initial breast and lymph node surgery rather than blood tests and scans?*

A That is correct. Most oncologists also order the type of routine blood tests that you would have as part of a general checkup. This blood test panel assesses the function of your bone marrow, liver, and kidneys. A chest X-ray for baseline purposes is reasonable as well. Special types of scans are generally reserved for patients with locally advanced breast cancer, stage III.

10

*

What Is Radiation Therapy?

Q *What is radiation therapy?*
A This is a form of cancer treatment that uses high energy X-rays (photons) delivered from a machine called a linear accelerator. The radiation is usually given daily except on weekends for about six weeks. Each treatment visit takes about fifteen minutes, although the initial treatment planning may take one to two hours.

Q *How do I know if I need radiation?*
A If you have an invasive breast cancer and are undergoing a lumpectomy, radiation therapy is <u>almost always given.</u> This will minimize the chance of breast cancer relapsing within the breast that has been operated on. Many studies on thousands of patients in North America and Europe show that breast conservation is equal to mastectomy in three important categories; control of cancer within the breast/chest area, freedom from relapse of cancer anywhere within the body, and overall survival. For successful breast conservation, it's essential that the lumpectomy clears the surgical margins of cancer. It's mandatory to have a rim of normal breast tissue between the cancer and the

the resection, ensuring that the cancer has been completely

in the treatment of DCIS, if a lumpectomy is performed, radiation therapy is usually given, except in cases of very small low grade DCIS that have been widely excised by the surgery.

Q *Do mastectomy patients ever need radiation?*

A Yes, there are certain situations following mastectomy where radiation can significantly reduce the chances of cancer returning within the mastectomy area and improve survival as well. The two most common situations needing radiation after mastectomy are either having a breast cancer larger than 5 cm in longest diameter, or having more than 3 lymph nodes containing cancer. Less common reasons for radiation after mastectomy are having a positive surgical margin (cancer at the edge of the mastectomy specimen), having a positive lymph node with capsular penetration (the cancer extends beyond the outer lining), or having lymphovascular invasion (involvement by cancer of the lymph channels within the breast).

Q *What are the side effects of radiation for breast cancer?*

A You won't actually feel the radiation during the actual treatment. Like taking a chest X-ray, there's no noticeable sensation from the radiation beam. The treatments can cause some tiredness but it's usually mild. During the last one to two weeks of treatment, the skin overlying the breast becomes pink like a sunburn and sometimes can temporarily blister. There may also be some tanning of the skin as the course of treatment ends. The older form of cobalt radiation caused much more severe skin problems compared to modern radiation techniques using a linear accelerator. With modern radiation, after one to two years the skin changes tend to be very mild and it can often be difficult to tell any difference compared to the opposite breast.

The radiation for breast cancer is carefully directed at an angle across the chest wall to avoid radiation exposure to internal body structures as much as possible. Therefore most of the beam passes through the breast without penetrating the entire chest cavity, although there is radiation effect on the ribs underlying the breast and also on the very

Radiation Therapy

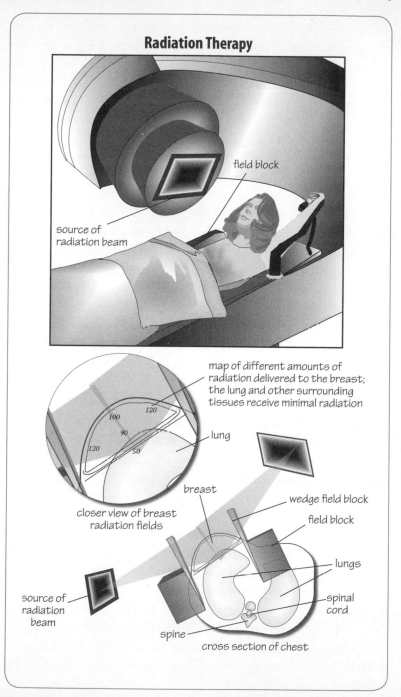

field block

source of
radiation beam

map of different amounts of
radiation delivered to the breast;
the lung and other surrounding
tissues receive minimal radiation

120
100
90
120
50

lung

breast

closer view of breast
radiation fields

wedge field block

field block

lungs

spinal
cord

source of
radiation
beam

spine

cross section of chest

front of the lung that is under the ribs. Over time, this can cause the ribs to be somewhat brittle and more susceptible to hairline fractures with severe bouts of coughing or a firm blow to the chest area. When this occurs, patients can develop pain from a hairline rib fracture that will heal on its own over one or two months. Some patients can also have soreness of the chest wall or muscles behind the breast as a result of radiation without having a rib fracture. Chest X-rays or CT scans can demonstrate scarring of the very front of the underlying lung but symptoms due to this are very rare.

ELLEN IS A psychiatric social worker in her mid-forties. She's full figured and has a fairly small right breast cancer. She's a good candidate for breast conservation but is fearful of radiation because her mother needed radiation for cancer of the uterus in the late 1960s and suffered from radiation damage to her pelvic area. Ellen doesn't want to have a mastectomy but because she is afraid of radiation therapy, she's leaning toward having one. I discuss the option of mastectomy with immediate reconstruction but also explain that modern radiation technology is vastly improved compared to her mother's time. Rather than make a decision now, I suggest that she have a consultation with the radiation oncologist to review her concerns.

Following her radiation consultation, Ellen meets with me several more times before eventually deciding, with trepidation, on breast conservation. She undergoes lumpectomy and sentinel node biopsy. After she is healed from surgery, she receives radiation. I'm seeing her for her post-radiation check and ask about her radiation experience.

"It was surprisingly good. Dr. Erickson and her staff were so professional and nice, I felt very comfortable and safe with them. They were very careful, making sure I was placed in just the right position for each treatment. Unlike you, they always ran on time, like clockwork. What do you do? Why aren't you ever on time? Anyway, they scheduled my treatments in the morning so that I could work. Toward the end, my breast hurt a little and became red and they gave me some creams to use. I never did blister."

As I examine her, I point out that she has had a very good cosmetic result. "Actually, now I like my right breast better than the left. It's fuller and has a better shape. My left one is droopy in comparison. Is there any chance I could have some radiation to the left one?"

I look at her face to see if she's joking and I can't tell. So I reply, "You've got some swelling of the breast from radiation, and after a year or two, it'll go away and the breast will look more like the one on the left. I'm very sure they won't agree to radiate your left breast."

I watch her for any indication of disappointment but again I can't read her. However, I'm pleased that she's pleased with how her treatment has worked out.

Q *I've had a lumpectomy. My surgeon removed the entire cancer and the margins are clear. I'm also receiving chemotherapy. Why do I also need radiation?*

A This is a very good question and is frequently asked. Studies of radiation therapy after lumpectomy show that when radiation is not given, there is a higher chance of cancer returning to the breast, often around the lumpectomy area. This can happen regardless of other treatments being given, including chemotherapy or hormonal therapy. When radiation is given after the lumpectomy margins are cleared, the risk of relapse within the breast is less than 5 to 7 percent, which also happens to be the risk of relapse within the scar of a mastectomy. There is concern that a recurrence within the breast may increase your chances of having cancer spread elsewhere, so that minimizing your recurrence risk by having radiation is prudent.

The need for radiation therapy after lumpectomy was recently reviewed by Dr. Vincent Vinh-Hung, a professor in Belgium, and Dr. Claire Verschraegen from the University of New Mexico. They analyzed 15 clinical trials containing almost 10,000 patients with invasive breast cancer. These trials compared patients who had only lumpectomy against patients who had lumpectomy and radiation. The patients who didn't receive radiation had triple the relapse rate within the breast and also had a slightly lower survival rate.

Having said that, there are recent studies of older patients (age seventy or more) undergoing lumpectomy only, without radiation, for small invasive cancers that have been widely excised. These studies demonstrate a fairly low recurrence risk (significantly less than 10 percent) within the breast. In one study reported by Dr. Kevin Hughes from Harvard, patients over the age of seventy with small ER positive cancers less than 2 cm received either lumpectomy alone or lumpectomy followed by radiation. When radiation wasn't given, the recurrence rate within the breast using only lumpectomy and Tamoxifen was 4 percent at five years, considered a fairly low number. However, even here, when radiation was added, the relapse rate within the breast fell from 4 percent to 1 percent.

In a note of caution regarding omitting radiation, Dr. Bernard Fisher and the NSABP had previously reported the results of a similarly designed study in 2002 showing a breast relapse rate of 16.5 percent at eight years when radiation wasn't used after lumpectomy. In Dr. Fisher's study all patients had cancers 1 cm or smaller, less breast cancer than Dr. Hughes's patients.

A relatively higher, but still fairly low risk of breast relapse may be acceptable in certain situations depending on the overall health and life expectancy of each individual patient. In older patients having other significant medical problems, consideration of omitting radiation therapy isn't unreasonable.

Q *Can breast radiation ever cause cancer?*

A This has been reported after radiation treatment for breast cancer but is very rare. After many years following radiation, extremely rare episodes of cancer within the radiation area can occur.

There is a higher risk of getting breast cancer after radiation exposure of the breast for treatment of Hodgkin's lymphoma. In treating Hodgkin's lymphoma, the breasts aren't the primary target of the radiation but unintentionally receive a moderate dose of radiation. The risk is primarily in women who had received radiation during teenage years. Women who received treatment when middle-aged have a significantly much lower risk.

Similarly, breast radiation for breast cancer is considered safe. As mentioned before, many studies show equal survival rates of breast conservation compared to mastectomy.

Q *So if I am advised that I can have breast radiation for my cancer instead of mastectomy, I can expect the same control rate within the breast area, the same overall cure rate of my cancer, and the same overall survival as if I had my breast removed with mastectomy?*

A Yes. That is why most patients choose to have breast conservation instead of mastectomy for breast cancer.

Q *Again, what are the reasons I might need a mastectomy instead of breast conservation?*

A The most common reason is having a large cancer relative to breast size, where a lumpectomy cannot be done with an acceptable cosmetic appearance. Sometimes a lumpectomy is attempted but the surgical margins cannot be cleared due to small extending fingers of residual cancer. When this happens, and there is enough breast volume remaining, a re-excision can be tried to clear margins. If the breast is large enough, multiple re-excisions can be tried but eventually if clear margins cannot be achieved, a mastectomy is needed.

Less common reasons for mastectomy are situations in which the cancer is multicentric. This term means that there are two or more cancers in different areas of the same breast. Sometimes mastectomy is recommended if the cancer is too close to the nipple, but even in this situation, breast conservation can still be performed by removing the nipple and having a plastic surgeon reconstruct it. This is done with very good cosmetic result by pulling up a section of skin to re-create the nipple contour and using tattoo to re-create the areola.

Q *If I have breast implants, can I still have radiation?*

A Yes, it's possible to have radiation for breast conservation with a breast implant in place. Although the cosmetic result can still be very good, on average it's not quite as good. There's a normal tendency for fibrosis or scarring around the implant, which is significantly increased with radiation. Some of my patients have also had breast implants put in place after lumpectomy and radiation for breast conservation. The healing process is slower because of radiation effect on breast tissue, but the cosmetic result can often be good. As discussed before, this shouldn't be confused with using an implant to reconstruct the breast following mastectomy with radiation. This is because a mastectomy removes all breast tissue and therefore an implant after mastectomy has only a layer of skin in front of it. The skin is stiffer and less pliable after radiation, and an implant in this setting tends to be too firm and uncomfortable.

Q *If radiation therapy doesn't work the first time, can it be given again to the same breast?*

A Usually not. One complete course of breast radiation for the purposes of breast conservation gives very close to the limit of radiation that the breast can tolerate safely. Excessive radiation causes the normal tissues of the breast to become permanently injured. There are rare circumstances where limited radiation can be given, but never at the doses required for breast conservation in breast cancer.

Q *What about other illnesses that might prevent me from getting breast radiation?*

A There are a few uncommon illnesses that require mastectomy because breast radiation cannot be given safely, such as scleroderma which is an inflammatory autoimmune disease affecting the skin. This disease causes the skin to become very tight and even uncomfortable. There is another autoimmune disease called systemic lupus. If the lupus is very active and there is a lot of skin inflammation, radiation therapy should be avoided and a mastectomy is the preferred treatment.

Q *What about the newer more limited radiation techniques like Mammosite because six weeks sounds like a long time?*

A There are more limited radiation regimens that have been studied, but the long-term control rates for these newer techniques are not known. A new device called the Mammosite, for limited local breast radiation, has been recently approved by the FDA for treating small breast cancers. This technique requires a lumpectomy followed by insertion of a balloon device through which radiation seeds are subsequently placed and removed twice daily for five days. It is important to note that only part of the breast is treated with this technique, the area immediately around the lumpectomy. The FDA, somewhat surprisingly, approved this device after studies with small numbers of patients and without long-term data.

The National Cancer Institute conducted a workshop at the end of 2002 evaluating all existing data on partial breast radiation. This is different from traditional breast radiation in which the entire breast receives treatment. This conference was lead by Dr. Norm Coleman, the Director of the Radiation Research Program at the National Cancer Institute. These experts recommended against the routine use of partial breast radiation in standard practice because of lack of sufficient data, but agreed that it should be studied in clinical trials.

The Mammosite technique may be appropriate in certain areas of the country where daily travel to a radiation therapy center is not feasible because of distance. However, I'm not currently recommending this technique to patients otherwise, because the radiation delivered by the Mammosite is to an area of about 1 cm from the device, not to the entire breast, and therefore it is in essence like having a large lumpectomy. This technique leaves a significant amount of breast untreated, and there is no long-term data on large numbers of patients demonstrating results equal to that of standard breast radiation. In addition, the Mammosite cannot be used for cancers close to the surface of the breast due to the potential for skin damage.

There will be several national studies of Mammosite for small breast cancers starting soon. It's anticipated that the early results will probably be acceptable. There is concern among many radiation oncologists about what the long-term results will be. The cosmetic results and control rate of cancer with standard breast radiation are so good that alternate techniques will need to be evaluated for over a decade in thousands of patients before they become standard alternatives.

11

※

What Is Adjuvant Therapy of Breast Cancer?

Q *What does the term adjuvant therapy mean?*

A The term adjuvant therapy refers to the use of cancer treatment in the absence of known disease. In breast cancer, this refers to the use of hormonal therapy and chemotherapy after breast surgery (postoperative treatment) to prevent the cancer from spreading or metastasizing.

There's also a term called neoadjuvant therapy referring to chemotherapy (or sometimes hormonal therapy) given prior to breast surgery, or in other words, preoperative treatment.

Q *Why is adjuvant therapy important?*

A The purpose of using adjuvant therapy in breast cancer is to improve cure rates mainly by preventing metastasis. Adjuvant therapy of breast cancer has been well established in numerous clinical trials throughout the world to reduce the risk of recurrence and death from breast cancer. For chemotherapy, the estimated benefit is about a 25 percent relative reduction in relapse rate. For hormonal therapy in receptor positive patients, the estimated benefit is about a 40 percent relative reduction in relapse rate. These numbers refer to reductions in relapse in all areas of the body, not just relapse within the breast or mastectomy area. It's important to keep in mind that chemotherapy can be used to reduce the recurrence risk in all breast cancer patients but hormonal therapy can only be helpful in patients with hormone receptors positive breast cancers.

Q *What is meant by a relative reduction in relapse rate?*
A This means that any breast cancer patient receiving the treatment will have a similar proportional lowering of her chances of having breast cancer recur regardless of her starting point.

As an example using chemotherapy, let's say you have, based on your cancer stage after surgery, an estimated recurrence risk over ten years of 20 percent. The addition of chemotherapy can reduce that risk to 15 percent. That reduction from 20 percent to 15 percent is a relative risk reduction of 25 percent. If this concept of relative risk reduction is confusing to you, it's also confusing to some experts. Essentially, adjuvant treatment offers a proportional benefit in preventing relapse and improving cure rate. The exact percentage point improvement resulting from treatment depends upon an individual patient's initial risk of metastasis, which can be estimated by initial cancer stage.

Q *Why is reducing breast cancer relapse important?*
A As I discussed in chapter 9, relapsing metastatic breast cancer is classified as stage IV breast cancer. With currently available treatments, we are unable to cure metastatic breast cancer. We are only able to cure patients with breast cancer limited to the breast and immediate lymph nodes, in other words stages I, II, and III. Therefore treatments that can reduce the relapse rate of breast cancer are essential in improving breast cancer cure and survival (see chapter 19).

Q *A 25 percent reduction in risk of recurrence by using chemotherapy doesn't sound like much. Why isn't the benefit higher than that?*
A With the use of modern chemotherapy, the benefit may very well be higher than 25 percent. The precise risk reduction number from chemotherapy is actually 23.5 percent. This number is based on a very extensive review of the world's clinical trial experience by Dr. Richard Peto and his team at Oxford University. He compared all

the patients who received chemotherapy against the patients who did not by combining all of the clinical trials.

What is significant regarding the effectiveness of adjuvant chemotherapy is the time frame that these clinical trials took place. Most of the clinical trials occurred in the late 1970s and early 1980s. At that time, neither patients nor their physicians were convinced that chemotherapy was helpful in improving breast cancer cure. Unlike today, because of what we now know, it was appropriate at that time to randomly select some patients to receive chemotherapy while others did not and to monitor their outcomes. Many patients on those trials received less than prescribed doses of their treatments due to significant side effects and the lack of conviction by patients and physicians that chemotherapy would help.

Today, modern chemotherapy is given with far fewer side effects as a result of many advances in controlling symptoms and reducing infection risk. I will discuss this further in chapters 16 and 17. In addition to being easier to receive, modern chemotherapy is also significantly more effective than treatments available in the late 1970s and early 1980s. Because current chemotherapy is both easier and more effective, both patients and physicians are now convinced that chemotherapy will help, so it's now uncommon for a patient to not receive adjuvant chemotherapy at fully prescribed doses.

For many reasons like these, it's very likely that modern chemotherapy will reduce the recurrence risk by a factor that is significantly greater than 25 percent. The exact degree of benefit can now never be proven, because it would be unethical to conduct a clinical trial in which some breast cancer patients who need chemotherapy would not be permitted to receive it. Because the benefit of chemotherapy is now proven, in all current clinical trials using adjuvant chemotherapy, the only question being tested in participating patients is the relative effectiveness of different chemotherapy programs, not the question of chemotherapy versus no chemotherapy.

DORIS IS SIXTY-THREE and soon to be a grandmother. She's looking forward to babysitting duties to help her daughter who will be a working mom. Doris is with her husband, Jim, an advertising executive. Several weeks ago she had a lumpectomy and sentinel node biopsy. The cancer was 2.6 cm and the sentinel node biopsy contained cancer on frozen section analysis by the pathologist in the operating room, so the surgeon performed an axillary dissection. She ended up with 3 of 15 positive nodes.

As I review with Doris and Jim the results of her surgery, I outline my recommendations for her to receive chemotherapy, followed by breast radiation, and an aromatase inhibitor for five years (she's ER positive).

Doris interrupts me and voices her unhappiness with my plan, "Wait a minute, Dr. Chan. I don't understand. Dr. Harrington said that he removed all the cancer and nothing was left behind. The margins were clear and the cancer was completely removed. I don't want any chemo. If I take chemo, I'm not going to be well enough to help Jenny with her baby. She needs me. If the surgeon got it all, why do I need chemo? My friend Elaine had the same surgery last year and her doctors told her she didn't need chemo."

I ask Doris how old Elaine is, how large her cancer was, and what the status of her lymph nodes was. It turns out that Elaine had a small cancer and was node negative.

I explain to Doris and Jim that we make chemotherapy recommendations based on estimated risk of cancer spread. Her friend, Elaine, had a lower stage cancer and therefore had a lower risk of relapse. Unfortunately, because of her 3 positive nodes, Doris has a significantly higher risk of relapse and needs chemotherapy to lower that risk.

I point out to Doris that it's likely, even on chemotherapy, that she'll feel well enough to help Jenny with her new baby. More importantly, by taking chemotherapy, Doris will have a higher chance of being well when her grandchild is two or three years old. And therefore, by taking chemotherapy she'll also have a better chance over time of being able to continue helping in the care of her grandchild.

Q *Are there also advances in adjuvant hormonal therapy?*

A Adjuvant hormonal therapy is also significantly improved, primarily for postmenopausal patients, as a result of newer medicines. Newer approaches to treating premenopausal patients are also currently under study. I'll review this in detail in chapter 12.

Q *Do all patients receive adjuvant hormonal therapy and chemotherapy?*

A Almost all patients with invasive breast cancer who are ER and/or PR positive (see chapter 6) receive adjuvant hormonal therapy because the treatments have a high margin of safety so the benefits are usually much greater than the risks. The more common side effects from hormonal therapy are generally minimal and major side effects are very infrequent.

The process of selecting which patients require chemotherapy is significantly more complicated because the side effects of chemotherapy are greater. Currently, the two most important factors determining whether chemotherapy is needed is lymph node status and tumor size. Most patients with lymph node involvement (node positive) and most patients with invasive cancers greater than 2 cm regardless of lymph nodes status are given chemotherapy if their health permits. There are some patients with negative nodes and cancers smaller than 2 cm who also receive chemotherapy. In these situations, the decision is often made based upon how close the cancer is to being 2 cm and also if the biomarker results are particularly unfavorable (chapter 6).

Patients with 1 to 2 cm cancers, negative nodes, who are ER and PR negative, cannot receive hormonal therapy and sometimes are considered for chemotherapy. This is often a difficult decision because the risks of relapse for smaller size cancers that are node negative are lower and therefore the potential benefit of chemotherapy is small.

Dr. Peter Ravdin at the University of Texas, San Antonio, has developed a remarkable computer program that helps calculate the risks of breast cancer relapse and the benefits of receiving adjuvant hormonal and chemotherapy based upon the results of clinical trials. This is a very helpful tool, particularly for patients who don't fall into one of the groups that clearly need adjuvant treatment. The program is available online. Patients should only access it with the help of their physician, because it is very important to input the data correctly to prevent erroneous results. Also, the information presented does require interpretation and explanation with a physician. You may ask your oncologist if this might be helpful for you.

12

＊

What Is Hormonal Therapy and Who Should Receive It?

Q *What is meant by hormonal therapy for breast cancer?*
A Hormonal therapy is different from chemotherapy. Hormonal therapy takes advantage of the relationship between the female hormones, estrogen and progesterone, and breast cancer growth. Many breast cancers have receptors for estrogen or progesterone and we call this being ER positive and PR positive. When a cancer is ER or PR positive (hormone receptor positive), it tends to depend on estrogen for growth and spread. In hormone receptor positive breast cancer, any change in estrogen level or activity can result in the cancer shrinking. Hormonal therapies can work by lowering levels of estrogen in the blood, or alternatively by preventing estrogen from attaching to the hormone receptors.

Q *How are ER and PR related?*
A These are both receptors that can be present in a breast cancer cell. They are tested for using special staining techniques performed on the breast biopsy specimen. The estrogen receptor (ER) is the site where estrogen attaches and the progesterone receptor (PR) is the site where

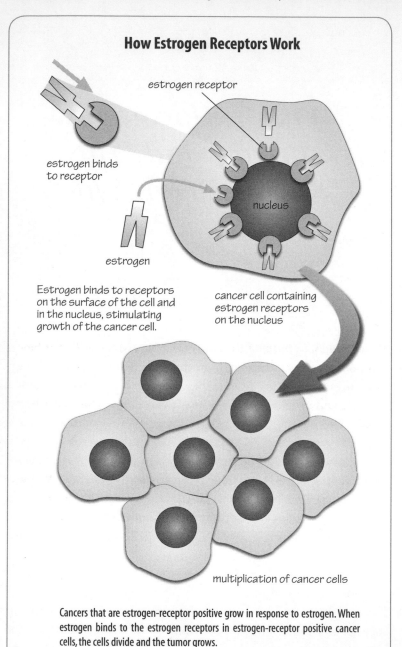

How Estrogen Receptors Work

estrogen receptor

estrogen binds
to receptor

nucleus

estrogen

Estrogen binds to receptors
on the surface of the cell and
in the nucleus, stimulating
growth of the cancer cell.

cancer cell containing
estrogen receptors
on the nucleus

multiplication of cancer cells

Cancers that are estrogen-receptor positive grow in response to estrogen. When
estrogen binds to the estrogen receptors in estrogen-receptor positive cancer
cells, the cells divide and the tumor grows.

progesterone attaches to the breast cancer cell. When estrogen attaches to these receptors, the growth of breast cancer is stimulated.

The likelihood of a cancer being receptor positive increases with increasing patient age. Sometimes the ER receptor is present and can bind estrogen but does not actually stimulate growth of the breast cancer. When this happens, hormonal therapy isn't effective and this explains why hormonal therapy does not work in every situation in which hormone receptors are positive. Usually when the ER receptor is active and stimulates cancer growth, it leads to the formation of the PR receptor.

Therefore patients with both ER and PR positivity have the best chance of responding to hormonal therapy. Studies suggest that if only one receptor is positive, then PR positivity may be more important than ER positivity. If both receptors are negative, hormonal therapy rarely helps.

Q *What is Tamoxifen?*
A Tamoxifen (brand name Nolvadex) is a once-a-day pill that blocks estrogen receptors. It does this by attaching to the receptor without activating it, and thereby prevents estrogen from attaching to the receptor. Tamoxifen belongs to a class of drugs called SERMs or selective estrogen receptor modulators. If you imagine the hormone receptor as being the ignition key to breast cancer growth, Tamoxifen has an effect like breaking the key off in the lock. You can't turn the broken key and another key, estrogen, can't get into the lock. Other drugs in this class include Fareston and Evista. Unlike some other hormone treatments that depend on menopausal status for effectiveness, Tamoxifen is active in both premenopausal and postmenopausal patients when hormone receptors are positive. This is an important point to keep in mind.

Q *When is Tamoxifen used?*
A Tamoxifen may be used for both adjuvant hormonal therapy and to treat metastatic breast cancer. It is used in the adjuvant setting (see chapter 11) following surgery in newly diagnosed patients who are hormone receptor positive. The standard length of time for use is five

years. Recent studies show that when Tamoxifen and chemotherapy are both being used, it's better to use chemotherapy first, followed by Tamoxifen rather than taking both at the same time. Taking chemotherapy and Tamoxifen together may result in Tamoxifen counteracting the effects of chemotherapy.

Tamoxifen is also used in metastatic breast cancer when the hormone receptors are positive. In metastatic disease, the length of time that Tamoxifen is used depends on how the cancer responds to treatment and varies from patient to patient. The length of response usually averages one to two years, although much longer control is sometimes possible.

Q *What are the main side effects of Tamoxifen?*

A Tamoxifen is a very safe drug and generally well tolerated. Like all medicines, there are downsides and risks, but the overall benefit in treating invasive breast cancer far outweighs the risks. Tamoxifen can infrequently cause mild nausea. It also blocks estrogen receptors within the brain, sometimes worsening postmenopausal symptoms (hot flashes). On rare occasions, Tamoxifen can cause depression or emotional imbalance. Because it's obviously very stressful to be receiving treatment for breast cancer, there may be many reasons for depression or emotional behavior to occur. When this happens, to test to see if Tamoxifen is responsible, I ask patients to stop taking it for several weeks to see if there is improvement. If the symptoms don't improve, then Tamoxifen is unlikely to be the cause.

Q *So far that doesn't sound too bad, but aren't there some serious side effects from Tamoxifen as well?*

A Yes, although they occur relatively infrequently. The more significant side effects didn't become known until Tamoxifen had been used in many thousands of patients over a period of about twenty years. About 1 to 1.5 percent of patients can develop blood clots in the veins of the legs, leading to pain and swelling. This is potentially dangerous because the clot can then travel to the lungs, leading to a pulmonary embolism, a serious problem.

There is also a small risk of developing cancer of the lining of the uterus, which is called the endometrium. This type of cancer is referred to as either uterine cancer or endometrial cancer. The risk is mainly in postmenopausal patients and is estimated to be increased from 1 percent to 2 percent by Tamoxifen. Both of these serious risks are considered low when compared to the benefits of improving cure rate and survival with Tamoxifen use in patients with invasive breast cancer. Whether the same holds true for use in DCIS is less certain because the level of danger from having DCIS is much less.

I caution my Tamoxifen patients to avoid dehydration and to stretch their legs frequently during long car or plane travel. They should also avoid crossing their legs while sitting, which puts pressure on the veins in the calf. I also ask them to see their gynecologist yearly and to undergo evaluation for any abnormal vaginal bleeding or spotting. Cancer of the uterus almost always results in some kind of abnormal vaginal bleeding or spotting. If attention is paid to this, the cancer is usually found early and studies show a very high cure rate with hysterectomy.

MARLENE IS THIRTY-EIGHT, a single mother, and a fitness fanatic. She's very health conscious, reads avidly about diet and exercise, takes multiple supplements, and adheres to a strict vegetarian diet. She had a lumpectomy for a 1.4 cm breast cancer with negative sentinel nodes. Her stage is T1N0 (stage I). She is ER and PR positive, Her2 negative.

I review with Marlene chemotherapy options, but she has a favorable breast cancer and is a borderline chemotherapy candidate. Because her situation is favorable, the benefit of chemotherapy is small, so although I explain that it's an option for her, I don't give her a recommendation to take it. However, I give her a strong recommendation to take Tamoxifen for five years and explain to her the overall benefits and the possible side effects.

Marlene is very upbeat and positive. "Look, Dr. Chan, I'm okay. I'm definitely not taking chemo and I don't think I want to take Tamoxifen. I've looked it up on the net, and Tamoxifen causes cancer of the uterus and blood clots. It doesn't sound like something I want to put into my body for five years. I really think I'll be fine. I don't like taking medications and I don't want those side effects. Is that okay?"

Not in my opinion. She does have a favorable breast cancer, but without Tamoxifen her chance of relapse over the next ten years is about 15 to 20 percent. She can cut her chances of relapse almost in half by taking Tamoxifen. Her chance of recurrence would be about 7 to 9 percent less, which in my mind, is a significant reduction.

The increased risk of cancer of the uterus from Tamoxifen is about 1 percent. Almost all cases are cured by hysterectomy if standard monitoring guidelines are followed. The risk of getting a blood clot is 1 to 1.5 percent. For Marlene, the potential benefits of taking Tamoxifen should significantly outweigh the risks.

Marlene's greatest danger is not the small chance of a major Tamoxifen side effect, but instead, a relapse of breast cancer that would make her stage IV and incurable. I ask her to strongly consider Tamoxifen and on her next follow-up visit she agrees to take it.

Q *I'm worried about the risk of cancer of the uterus. Are there any screening tests that should be performed?*

A There are no routine screening tests currently recommended. In premenopausal patients, the lining of the uterus is lost as part of the blood flow during a menstrual period so that the risk of uterine cancer is much lower compared to postmenopausal women. Keep in mind that in postmenopausal women, the normal risk of uterine cancer is fairly low, about 1 percent over a period of ten years. Tamoxifen increases this risk to about 2 percent, so the chance of getting uterine cancer from Tamoxifen is still fairly low. If abnormal vaginal bleeding is promptly evaluated by a gynecologist, cancer is usually found early and hysterectomy results in a very high cure rate. It's currently recommended that ultrasounds of the uterus or endometrial biopsies (biopsies of the lining of the uterus) only be performed if there is abnormal vaginal spotting or bleeding rather than on a routine yearly basis.

Q *Aside from reducing breast cancer recurrence, are there other benefits to Tamoxifen?*

A An important added benefit is a reduction in the risk of getting a breast cancer in the opposite breast. On average, a newly diagnosed breast cancer patient has a risk of developing a breast cancer in the opposite breast of about 0.75 percent per year (three-fourths of one percent per year). This means that over ten years, the risk of getting a new cancer in the opposite breast is 7.5 percent. Tamoxifen will reduce this risk roughly in half. Tamoxifen also acts as a weak estrogen on bones so that osteoporosis (softening of bones) is reduced. A related SERM, Evista, is often used to treat osteoporosis and has also been shown to significantly reduce the risk of breast cancer in women taking it for osteoporosis.

Q *What are aromatase inhibitors?*

A Aromatase inhibitors are often abbreviated as AIs. There are three medications in this group and they all come in pill form and are taken once a day. They are effective only in postmenopausal patients. It's very important to note that they don't work in premenopausal patients. The three drugs are anastrozole (Arimidex), letrozole (Femara), and exemestane (Aromasin). They have an effect by stopping an enzyme called aromatase, which makes small amounts of estrogen in post-menopausal patients. This causes a further lowering of already low estrogen levels. However, in premenopausal and even perimenopausal patients (women close to menopause), the ovaries make such high levels of estrogen that the aromatase inhibitors don't significantly affect estrogen levels and therefore can't be used.

If you imagine estrogen as being like fuel for breast cancer, after menopause the fuel tank is already low. The action of aromatase inhibitors is to basically empty the tank. Before menopause, the tank is so full that the small leak caused by the aromatase inhibitors doesn't have much effect.

Q *Who should receive aromatase inhibitors?*

A AIs are now becoming the hormonal therapy of first choice in the adjuvant and metastatic setting in patients who are clearly postmeno-pausal. A number of important recent adjuvant studies all showed slight improvement over Tamoxifen. Keep in mind that the AIs can only be used in postmenopausal patients who are ER or PR positive.

The AI clinical studies all vary somewhat in how the aromatase inhibitor was used. The most well known study is the ATAC trial,

How Tamoxifen Works

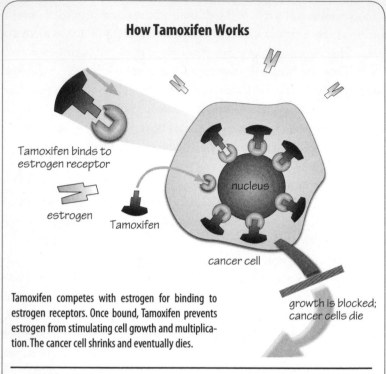

Tamoxifen binds to estrogen receptor

estrogen

Tamoxifen

nucleus

cancer cell

growth is blocked; cancer cells die

Tamoxifen competes with estrogen for binding to estrogen receptors. Once bound, Tamoxifen prevents estrogen from stimulating cell growth and multiplication. The cancer cell shrinks and eventually dies.

How Aromatase Inhibitors Work

androgen

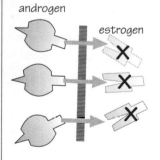

estrogen

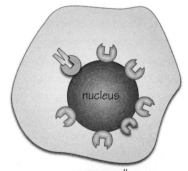

nucleus

cancer cell

aromatase inhibitors block production of estrogens

The body's fat, muscles, and adrenal glands make androgen-like hormones that are made into estrogen by an enzyme called aromatase. In postmenopausal patients, aromatase inhibitors are used to block that enzyme and prevent estrogen from being made. This prevents tumor growth.

which compared 5 years of Tamoxifen to 5 years of Arimidex. Arimidex was more effective than Tamoxifen in preventing relapse of breast cancer. Recently, a similar trial using Femara compared to Tamoxifen showed similar results. A trial from Canada, the MA17, reported that adding Femara following the standard 5 years of Tamoxifen was better than taking 5 years of Tamoxifen alone. The IES trial from Europe showed that after 2 or 3 years of Tamoxifen, switching to Aromasin to complete a total of 5 years of combined hormonal therapy was more effective than just taking Tamoxifen for 5 years.

Therefore, in receptor positive postmenopausal patients, the use of AIs has advantage over Tamoxifen. Like Tamoxifen, the AIs also reduce the risk of breast cancer in the opposite breast. It must be re-emphasized that AIs are not active in premenopausal or even perimenopausal patients. If a patient is premenopausal and taking chemotherapy for newly diagnosed breast cancer, Tamoxifen should be used initially after chemotherapy until it is certain that the menstrual periods have stopped because sometimes they resume months after the patient finishes chemotherapy. Only when it is certain that a patient is postmenopausal (which can be confirmed by blood tests of hormone levels) should a switch to an aromatase inhibitor be considered.

Q *Can you tell me more about the ATAC trial using Arimidex?*

A This was the first clinical trial that showed superiority of an aromatase inhibitor over Tamoxifen in newly diagnosed receptor positive postmenopausal breast cancer patients. It needs to be emphasized that the patients were all postmenopausal. The trial had three treatment groups. One group received Tamoxifen for 5 years, a second group received Arimidex for 5 years, and a third group received both. Initial reports suggested and subsequent analysis has confirmed that women receiving Arimidex had a lower relapse rate than those receiving Tamoxifen. Also women on Arimidex overall felt better with lower daily side effects and lower risks of blood clots and cancer of the uterus, which predictably occurred infrequently in women on Tamoxifen. Interestingly, the women receiving both Tamoxifen and Arimidex together had a relapse rate similar to the Tamoxifen only group. The reason for this is unclear.

Q *Do other aromatase inhibitors have similar effectiveness?*

A As I'll discuss below, there are a number of different studies that evaluate various aromatase inhibitors. For example, although ATAC was the first AI study to be reported, recently a similar study using Femara, the BIG1–98 trial, demonstrated similar benefits with 5 years of Femara compared to 5 years of Tamoxifen.

Rather than confusion about the various studies comparing different AIs, I think the take-home lesson should be that the current treatment of hormone receptor positive postmenopausal breast cancer patients should generally incorporate the use of an aromatase inhibitor, either in place of Tamoxifen or following some period of Tamoxifen use. Again it's essential to note that aromatase inhibitors will not work in premenopausal patients.

Q *Can you tell me more about the MA 17 trial using Femara?*

A This trial was conducted in Canada. All postmenopausal women with newly diagnosed receptor positive breast cancer initially received 5 years of Tamoxifen. When the 5 years of Tamoxifen were completed, some women were selected to receive Femara, while other women received no further hormonal therapy. Those women who received Femara after Tamoxifen had a lower recurrence rate than the women receiving only Tamoxifen. The amount of improvement by adding Femara is similar to the amount of improvement demonstrated by using Arimidex on the ATAC trial.

Q *Can you tell me more about the IES trial using Aromasin?*

A This trial was conducted in Europe. Postmenopausal women with newly diagnosed receptor positive breast cancer were initially started on Tamoxifen. After 2 to 3 years of Tamoxifen use, some of the women were randomly switched to Aromasin to complete 5 years total of hormonal therapy. For example, if a woman took 3 years of Tamoxifen, she then received 2 years of Aromasin. The women who were switched to Aromasin had a lower relapse rate than the women who stayed on Tamoxifen. As is a familiar theme, the degree of improvement from using Aromasin was similar to that shown by using Arimidex on the ATAC trial.

Q *Do aromatase inhibitors have side effects?*

A They have not been in use as long as Tamoxifen, nor in nearly as many patients, so the side effect profiles are still being developed. However, aromatase inhibitors generally seem to have fewer overall side effects than Tamoxifen. A small number of patients can get mild nausea or diarrhea. If this occurs, the symptoms often improve with continued use. Postmenopausal symptoms such as hot flashes tend to be less common and less severe than with Tamoxifen. Compared to Tamoxifen, there is probably no increased risk of blood clots in the legs and probably no increased risk of cancer of the uterus. However the AIs do seem to have a higher risk of osteoporosis (softening of the bones) and measures should be taken to counteract that. These include monitoring bone density by X-ray and taking a bisphosphonate medication which improves bone density, such as Fosamax or Actonel. Alternative measures include taking vitamin D, calcium supplements, and participating in weight bearing exercise. In general, the AIs are safe and well tolerated. They are significantly more expensive than Tamoxifen, even more so if Fosamax or Actonel are added to protect the bones. More data on less frequent side effects will be available as AIs become more frequently used.

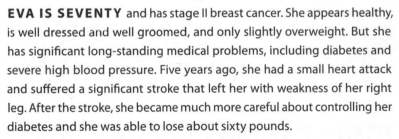

EVA IS SEVENTY and has stage II breast cancer. She appears healthy, is well dressed and well groomed, and only slightly overweight. But she has significant long-standing medical problems, including diabetes and severe high blood pressure. Five years ago, she had a small heart attack and suffered a significant stroke that left her with weakness of her right leg. After the stroke, she became much more careful about controlling her diabetes and she was able to lose about sixty pounds.

Eva needed a mastectomy with sentinel node biopsy. Two of the three sentinel nodes were positive. She then had a second operation for an axillary dissection and twelve more nodes were negative. Because of her other health problems, she was a borderline candidate for chemotherapy. I recommended to Eva that she take an aromatase inhibitor without chemotherapy and she agreed.

Seeing her after several months of taking the medication, I ask her how she feels. "Well, actually I feel pretty good. I have some mild hot flashes. I do feel a little more achy, but I can't really tell if it's the medicine or I'm just getting older. As you instructed, I took the Arimidex for a month and then added the Actonel. I have a hard time remembering to take the Actonel because I'm only taking it once a week. But I feel okay except for the soreness and it's mostly in my joints. Is it the medicine or my age?"

It's probably some of each, because she did have similar but milder symptoms before starting the treatment. Eva agrees that it's a small price to pay for cutting her recurrence risk by almost half and she wants to stay on the hormonal therapy.

Q *Aromatase inhibitors are never used in premenopausal patients?*

A Never say never. Premenopausal patients can receive AIs if something is medically done to make the premenopausal patient become post-menopausal. This can be accomplished by surgically removing the ovaries, which often can be performed with a laparoscope. The same effect can result from using a medication that can stop the ovaries from making estrogen. There are two medications that can do this, Depolupron and Zoladex. These medications are given by injection and stop the ovaries from making estrogen, effectively changing a patient from being premenopausal to being postmenopausal. Unlike removing the ovaries surgically, the effect is temporary and stops when the medication in discontinued. This change allows the use of aromatase inhibitors in younger patients.

Q *What is Faslodex?*

A This is a new type of hormonal therapy with the generic name of fulvestrant. Faslodex is given by injection into the muscle once a month. The drug causes the estrogen receptor to degrade. If you again imagine estrogen being a key and the estrogen receptor being the lock, Faslodex basically breaks the lock so that the key will not work. Although Faslodex has been tested in postmenopausal patients, theoretically it should have activity in all patients who are receptor positive, regardless of menopause status. Right now it is approved only for use in treating metastatic disease.

Q *What is Megace?*

A This is a progesterone pill, medroxyprogesterone, that is used in treating metastatic breast cancer. Prior to the approval of aromatase inhibitors, Megace was frequently used as a second line hormonal therapy after Tamoxifen. Now it is used after the AIs as a third or fourth line treatment in patients who are hormone receptor positive and have metastatic disease. The main problem with Megace is that it needs to be taken four times daily and has a side effect of stimulating hunger so that significant weight gain is a big problem. The weight gain, if unchecked, can be 2 to 3 pounds a month or about 25 pounds a year. Patients on Megace are cautioned not to eat just because they're hungry because they're hungry most of the time.

Q *What is the bottom line when using hormonal therapy to prevent breast cancer recurrence following surgery?*

A Either the estrogen or progesterone receptor needs to be positive. Having both hormone receptors being positive is better than just having just one. Having higher levels of receptors are better than lower levels. For adjuvant treatment of premenopausal women, the standard is Tamoxifen. For adjuvant treatment of postmenopausal women, the standard has changed to aromatase inhibitors. At this time there doesn't seem to be a difference in effectiveness or side effects between the three AIs, Arimidex, Aromasin, and Femara. Postmenopausal patients on Tamoxifen can either change to an AI and complete 5 years of therapy, or add an AI after 5 years of Tamoxifen. Which strategy is better is currently unknown, but either is acceptable.

13

✳

What Is Chemotherapy and Do I Need It?

Q *What is chemotherapy?*

A Chemotherapy refers to medicines that directly kill cancer cells by interfering with their ability to replicate. The majority of chemotherapy drugs are given intravenously, meaning into the veins. There are many different chemotherapy drugs in cancer treatment, and at least ten drugs that have some effectiveness in treating breast cancer. However, when newly diagnosed patients are being treated with adjuvant chemotherapy to prevent relapse, only a few drugs, the most active ones, are commonly used.

Q *What is the concept of adjuvant chemotherapy?*

A As I discussed in chapter 11, chemotherapy is frequently given after breast surgery to prevent recurrence. The surgery can be either lumpectomy or mastectomy. Surgery only treats the cancer within the breast. The danger from breast cancer is its potential to spread (metastasize). In the vast majority of newly diagnosed breast cancer patients, the currently available tests, whether it's blood work or scans (CT, MRI, PET), cannot confirm whether or not small undetectable amounts of cancer have spread.

Adjuvant treatment is the term used when chemotherapy is given in this situation, to treat potential cancer spread without having actual proof of spread. If metastatic cancer exists, using chemotherapy at this time allows treatment when there is the least amount of spreading cancer. What makes adjuvant chemotherapy decisions difficult is the potential side effects of treatment and the inability to know with certainty in any individual patient whether or not she has microscopic metastasis.

However, waiting and reserving chemotherapy until relapsing metastatic breast is established isn't reasonable because that situation cannot currently be cured with available treatments (see chapter 21). Many major clinical trials confirm that giving chemotherapy right after surgery improves breast cancer cure rates. The treatment is essentially being used in a preventative fashion and all patients in the appropriate risk groups are treated without the specific knowledge of knowing whether or not they are cancer free at the time.

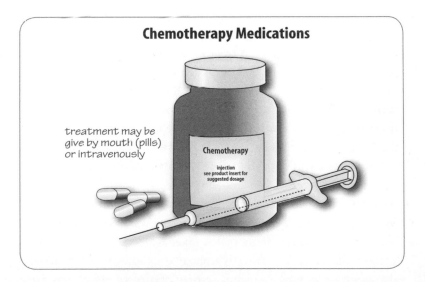

Chemotherapy Medications

treatment may be give by mouth (pills) or intravenously

Chemotherapy

injection
see product insert for
suggested dosage

Q *What is neoadjuvant chemotherapy?*
A This term refers to chemotherapy given before, instead of after, breast surgery. This is also called preoperative chemotherapy. Chemotherapy before surgery is usually considered when treating a larger cancer.

is to use chemotherapy to shrink the cancer and permit a
ıy rather than a mastectomy while also reducing the risk
ıis. This strategy has become very common over the past
five years and is often successful in allowing breast conservation and
reducing the need for mastectomy.

A number of studies have demonstrated a higher rate of breast conservation so that preoperative chemotherapy is often considered when
the breast cancer is large for women who wish to avoid a mastectomy.
Using chemotherapy earlier in the sequence of treatments doesn't
improve the cure rate compared to using chemotherapy after surgery,
but does decrease the need for mastectomy. It is clearly established
with a number of clinical trials that chemotherapy has equal cure rates
when given either before or after surgery.

Q *What are the commonly used chemotherapy drugs in adjuvant
programs?*

A There are four main classes of drugs combined in various combinations
in adjuvant chemotherapy programs. In treating metastatic breast
cancer, there are many more drugs available because the strategy of
chemotherapy use differs in treating early breast cancer as opposed
to metastatic breast cancer. For details see chapters 11 and 22.

The first class of drugs used for adjuvant treatment is alkylators that
work by directly binding to DNA and preventing duplication. The
main drug in this class is Cytoxan (cyclophosphamide). The second
class of drugs is anthracyclines that initially were made by fungi and
also inhibit DNA duplication. The two main drugs in this group are
Adriamycin (doxorubicin) and Ellence (epirubicin). The third most
commonly used class is the taxanes, drugs made from the western yew
tree, which stop cell division by disrupting the microtubule system
needed to support cell division. The taxanes are Taxol (paclitaxel) and
Taxotere (docetaxel). The fourth group of drugs used is antimetabolites
that work by stopping enzyme activity needed to make new DNA.
The drugs in this group are Methotrexate and Flourouracil.

It's important for you to know the names of the chemotherapy
drugs because different chemotherapy programs contain different
drug combinations. Although chemotherapy drugs have some com-

mon side effects, each drug also has individual side effects that need to be monitored.

Q *How can I conceptualize the way that chemotherapy works to destroy breast cancer?*

A If you can imagine the growth of a cancer like constructing a building, the alkylators and anthracyclines would work by covering up the blueprint so that the plans can't be implemented. The taxanes would prevent the workers from erecting the frame. The antimetobolites would prevent the delivery of building materials. The different types of chemotherapy permit the cancer to be attacked in different ways.

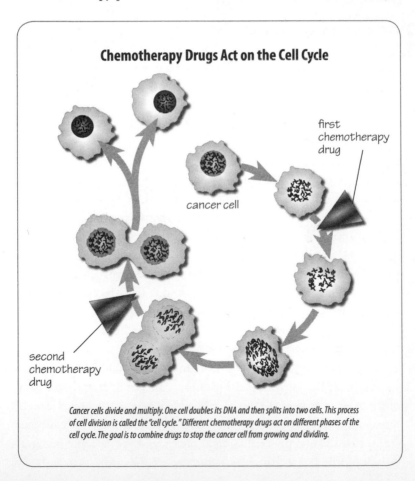

Chemotherapy Drugs Act on the Cell Cycle

first chemotherapy drug

cancer cell

second chemotherapy drug

Cancer cells divide and multiply. One cell doubles its DNA and then splits into two cells. This process of cell division is called the "cell cycle." Different chemotherapy drugs act on different phases of the cell cycle. The goal is to combine drugs to stop the cancer cell from growing and dividing.

Q *How is it that chemotherapy really works?*
A The ultimate effect of all chemotherapy drugs is to prevent cancer cell division, a very complicated process requiring many steps. Each step can potentially be disrupted. Our bodies normally heal and repair themselves by replacing existing cells with new ones. This occurs through a process called cell division in which the DNA duplicates itself, and eventually results in duplication of all the components making up a cell. By this process, one cell can become two, two can become four, and so on. This is also the way that cancer cells grow. Chemotherapy drugs, through many different mechanisms, prevent cell division and cause the cancer to die.

Q *Why does chemotherapy cause side effects?*
A Many of the common side effects of chemotherapy are a result of the nondiscriminating nature of chemotherapy. The drugs used are non-specific and do not completely distinguish between cancer cells and normal cells. Chemotherapy is effective because cancer cells typically grow much faster than normal cells. Therefore it is to be hoped that the damage to the cancer is beyond repair, while normal cells that are less affected can repair over time.

The fastest growing cells in our bodies are those in the bone marrow, in the hair follicles, and in the lining of the gastrointestinal tract. This is why the most common side effects of breast cancer chemotherapy include lowered blood counts and hair loss. These are temporary side effects and improve when chemotherapy is completed. Contrary to popular belief, the nausea that can be associated with chemotherapy is due to stimulation of receptors in the brain. These receptors perceive the chemotherapy as a toxin and cause a nausea reflex.

Q *How are the chemotherapy drugs selected for use?*
A This occurs through extensive testing in clinical trials. More national resources are currently devoted to breast cancer research than to any other type of cancer. Many of the advancements in breast cancer research are due to patients like yourself who enroll in a National Cancer Institute supported clinical breast cancer trial. The researchers select different treatments that are believed by experts to be fairly

equivalent in benefit. A computer randomly selects which regimen is given to each patient, and the results are analyzed over many years. For a treatment to be proven superior, it must reach a degree of significance that statisticians calculate does not reflect just random chance. Each clinical trial can cost many tens of millions of dollars to conduct. Oncologists don't accept a treatment as being the proven best until it is tested in this manner. This type of study is called a phase 3 study, which I'll discuss in more detail in chapter 22.

Q *What about chemotherapy sensitivity assays to select the chemotherapy specifically for me and my individual breast cancer?*

A This is an appealing strategy, but unfortunately has been a disappointing test. When chemotherapy assays were first developed over twenty years ago, there was hope that chemotherapy could be selected like antibiotics. A patient's cancer cells would be grown in test tubes. Chemotherapy drugs would be placed into the different test tubes and whichever drug showed the best cancer kill would be selected for use.

These types of assays have been evaluated in clinical trials, including trials conducted by the National Cancer Institute, and unfortunately were found to be fairly ineffective for chemotherapy selection. There are a number of reasons for this. Cancer growth often depends on multiple factors, including a very complicated support system from surrounding non-cancer cells that can't be replicated in a test tube. Many chemotherapy drugs are inactive until metabolized (changed by the body), a process that can take many steps with many metabolites possibly having different ways of stopping cancer growth.

The utility of chemotherapy sensitivity assays was recently reviewed by two study groups and reported in 2004, one led by Dr. David Samson for Blue Cross and Blue Shield, and a second led by Dr. Deborah Schrag for the American Society of Clinical Oncology (ASCO, our national oncology organization). Both groups came to the same conclusion based on existing clinical trials that generally show these tests as ineffective. These study groups confirmed what the oncology centers learned by experience, that the routine use of chemotherapy sensitivity assays cannot be recommended.

Unfortunately, the fairly simplified technique of chemotherapy assays is unable to replicate the very complex interaction between cancer cells and chemotherapy that actually occurs within the body. In the future, it is likely that chemotherapy selection will be made more individually than is currently the case but it will be based on genomic and proteomic tests. Each cancer patient will have specific tests of her cancer to analyze its genetic makeup (genomic testing) and to identify specific proteins which that cancer produces in order to grow (proteomic testing). An analysis of these factors will permit individualized selection of chemotherapy and targeted therapy known to be most effective for specific combinations of genetic patterns and protein growth factors. Many clinical trials using genomic and proteomic tests are already underway in breast cancer with preliminary data that is very promising because these tests truly get to the essence of what makes an individual's cancer different.

Q; *How do I know if I need chemotherapy?*

A This decision is made in partnership with your oncologist and involves a complex calculation of your risk of relapse as I discussed in chapter 11.

Estimated Ten-Year Disease-Free Survival in Breast Cancer Patients Treated ONLY with Breast Conservation or Mastectomy

Positive Nodes	Size of Cancer					
	<1 cm	1–2 cm	2–3 cm	3–4 cm	4–5 cm	>5 cm
0	90%	81%	75%	69%	63%	56%
1–3	60%	56%	50%	47%	42%	37%
4–6	46%	42%	38%	35%	31%	27%
7–9	38%	32%	29%	26%	21%	18%
>9	22%	19%	17%	16%	14%	13%

This table was developed by Dr. Loprinzi at the May Clinic and based on estimates made by 10 national breast cancer experts. The table can be used to determine the need for adjuvant hormonal and adjuvant chemotherapy.

In general, if you're healthy, and have breast cancer that has gone into lymph nodes or if your breast cancer is 2 cm in size or greater, you should be considered for chemotherapy. This recommendation is based upon a thorough review of the existing clinical trials data by the National Institutes of Health Consensus Conference. If you have no lymph node involvement but have a cancer between 1 and 2 cm, chemotherapy may be considered, depending on other biological markers such as ER,PR, Her2, and Ki-67. When hormone receptors are negative, hormonal therapy cannot be used so chemotherapy is the only option to address the potential of spreading breast cancer. If you have a very small invasive cancer, the benefit of taking chemotherapy is usually too small to warrant its use. Chemotherapy is never used to treat DCIS because the risk of spread is negligible.

DEBRA IS FORTY-FOUR, an accountant, single, and without children. She is slim, athletic, and competes in masters swimming. She has a 1.6 cm breast cancer that is completely removed by lumpectomy with negative sentinel nodes. She is ER and PR positive, Her2 negative. In addition to radiation, I recommend that she take Tamoxifen because she is premenopausal.

I also review with Debra the option of chemotherapy. Without it, her chance of recurrence over the next ten years is 10 to 15 percent. By taking chemo, her recurrence rate would drop to 6 to 10 percent, a reduction of about one-third. The benefit isn't large, but it's also not insignificant. I don't give Debra a specific recommendation for chemotherapy because situations like this require a balanced discussion of the benefits and risks of treatment. I review these with her and ask her to think about it. We arrange another appointment to make a treatment decision.

By her next visit, she has made her decision. "Dr. Chan, I've thought long and hard about chemo. I've talked to my sister and close friends. And I've decided not to take it. Maybe it's a selfish decision but I don't know any other way to make it. You see, I'm single and I don't have kids or anyone I need to take care of. I'm really happy with my life right now, and I don't want to interrupt work or stop swimming and competing. If I've got this right, chemo will help me by about 4 to 5 percent. That means that there's

6 percent chance it wouldn't make a difference for me. Did I
correctly?" I nod yes. "That's just not a big enough difference
receive it. Don't you agree?"

Given her personal circumstances and her low risk of recurrence,
I believe she's thought it through correctly. For Debra, it's the right
decision.

Q *Do all patients get the same kind of chemotherapy?*

A Actually no, although there are only a few commonly used standard
programs. The specific chemotherapy program is usually selected
based upon your estimated risk of relapse. Again, this risk can
be estimated by using mainly lymph node status and tumor size,
and then to a much lesser extent, the biomarkers such as ER, PR,
Her2, and Ki-67. Some patients have a low to moderate relapse risk
and can be treated with chemotherapy regimens that have lower
side effects. Patients with significant lymph node involvement or
larger breast cancers need more aggressive chemotherapy in order
to be cured.

Q *Will adjuvant chemotherapy definitely improve my cure rate?*

A Studies using adjuvant chemotherapy involving tens of thousands of breast cancer patients over the past twenty-five years
have established improvement in breast cancer cure rates. As I
discussed in chapter 11, the use of adjuvant chemotherapy will
lower your relapse rate by a factor of at least 25 percent. During
these initial chemotherapy trials, chemotherapy effectiveness was
probably underestimated, because in the past the treatments had
very significant side effects and many patients couldn't complete
the planned treatment.

However with major advances in controlling nausea and
chemotherapy-related blood problems, and with the introduction of better chemotherapy drugs, the chemotherapy regimens
have become much more effective. How much better, we'll never
know for sure because it would be unethical to perform a clinical trial today, which compares a group of women who receive

chemotherapy against a group of women who don't, since the overall effectiveness of chemotherapy is well established.

Q *What if I choose to wait, and take chemotherapy only if my cancer comes back?*

A Many patients ask me this question and it's a very good question. Unfortunately, the answer is that if breast cancer returns anywhere outside of the breast area, such as the lungs or liver, it is classified as stage IV or metastatic disease. Given the currently available treatments, metastatic breast cancer is not curable. That's why the initial decision to receive or not receive adjuvant chemotherapy is so important.

This doesn't mean that every new breast cancer patient should receive chemotherapy. Chemotherapy isn't used in patients with DCIS. In patients with small invasive cancers and negative lymph nodes, chemotherapy is often not recommended, particularly if hormone receptors are positive and hormonal therapy can be used. If the risk of recurrence is estimated to be low, usually chemotherapy is not justified.

RHONDA IS TWENTY-NINE, engaged to a physician, and has high grade DCIS. The estimated size on mammogram is 3 cm. Her breasts are small and she undergoes mastectomy with sentinel node biopsy. The nodes are normal except for two cancer cells that are seen only by the use of special stain (cytokeratin). She then has an axillary dissection with fifteen negative nodes.

Rhonda's sister had breast cancer several years ago at the age of thirty-nine. She had three positive nodes, took chemotherapy, and is doing well. Rhonda is very afraid of recurrence and wants chemotherapy.

I explain to her and her fiancé, a dermatology resident, that DCIS is noninvasive, is not considered life threatening, and shouldn't metastasize. The significance of the two cells within the node is very unclear. Rather than indicating a biologic tendency for her DCIS to spread, the cells could just as well have been dislodged from the DCIS by the core needle biopsy. I also review with them that the meaning of cancer cells in a sentinel node biopsy for DCIS is very unclear. A meticulous review by the pathologist of the mastectomy specimen didn't show any invasive cancer, only DCIS.

Rhonda's cure rate without chemotherapy should be close to 100 percent. Although I understand Rhonda's fear, I feel that she is much more likely to have toxicity from chemotherapy than benefit. I explain to them why in her particular case, I'm not in favor of chemotherapy and I wouldn't be comfortable giving it to her.

Her fiancé listens intently, nodding his head, from time to time. He then turns to her, "I understand what Dr. Chan is saying and he's probably right. But I know how you feel about this. Whatever you decide is fine."

Rhonda wants chemotherapy. "I really do understand everything you said, and it makes perfect sense to me based on the things I've read and what others have told me. Nonetheless, I can't stop thinking about those two cancer cells in that node and the possibility that there might be others somewhere else. What if they weren't put there by the biopsy? I know it's crazy but if there's a one-tenth of 1 percent chance that it'll help me, I want the strongest chemotherapy."

I disagree with her decision. In Rhonda's situation, the risks of chemotherapy significantly outweigh the benefits. She decides to change doctors and gets chemotherapy.

It doesn't mean that I'm right and she's wrong, or the other way around. What this illustrates is that not every doctor and patient are a good match.

☀

Q *What are the common chemotherapy regimens?*

A If patients have smaller cancers and negative lymph nodes, a regimen called CMF is often given for 6 months. CMF is one the oldest regimens and was developed by Dr. Gianni Bonadonna, the director of the National Cancer Institute, Italy. It consists of Cytoxan, Methotrexate, and Flourouracil. CMF tends to cause less nausea and hair loss than the other regimens commonly used. Studies have shown that a shorter regimen called AC (Adriamycin and Cytoxan) given for 3 months (4 treatments given 3 weeks apart) is as effective as CMF but causes more nausea and hair loss.

A more aggressive regimen is FAC or FEC for 6 treatments given 3 weeks apart. FAC contains Flourouracil, Adriamycin and Cytoxan while FEC substitutes Ellence for Adriamycin. FEC is widely used in Canada and Europe. Another aggressive chemotherapy regimen frequently used in the United States is AC for 3 months followed by a taxane, either Taxol or Taxotere, for 3 months. This is often referred to as AC followed by T or ACT. Again the treatments are given every 3 weeks. These more aggressive regimens are more active against breast cancer but also have potential for more side effects and therefore can be somewhat more difficult to receive.

Q *What is dose-dense chemotherapy?*
A This refers to chemotherapy given at standard doses in a sequential fashion with the time in between treatments compressed. The concept isn't new but the benefit is only recently proven. In standard regimens, the chemotherapy is given every 3 weeks. However, recent studies show that decreasing the time between treatments

Chemotherapy Programs for Node Positive Patients

Program	Week																						
	1	2	3	4	5	6	7	8	9	10	11	12	13	14	15	16	17	18	19	20	21	22	23
FEC																							
Flourouracil	✔			✔			✔			✔			✔			✔							
Ellence	✔			✔			✔			✔			✔			✔							
Cytoxan	✔			✔			✔			✔			✔			✔							
TAC																							
Taxotere	✔			✔			✔			✔			✔			✔							
Adriamycin	✔			✔			✔			✔			✔			✔							
Cytoxan	✔			✔			✔			✔			✔			✔							
AC->Taxotere																							
Adriamycin	✔			✔			✔			✔													
Cytoxan	✔			✔			✔			✔													
Taxotere													✔			✔			✔			✔	
Dose Dense AC->Taxol																							
Adriamycin	✔		✔		✔		✔																
Cytoxan	✔		✔		✔		✔																
Taxol									✔		✔		✔		✔								
Dose Dense ATC																							
Adriamycin	✔		✔		✔		✔																
Taxol									✔		✔		✔		✔								
Cytoxan																	✔		✔		✔		✔

improves the effectiveness of the chemotherapy. This concept was developed by Drs. Larry Norton, Clifford Hudis, and their team at Memorial Sloan-Kettering Cancer Center in New York. An example of dose-dense chemotherapy is to use AC followed by T every 2 weeks rather than every 3 weeks. This type of scheduling is possible because of the development of bone marrow growth factors that speed the recovery of blood counts.

Q *What is Herceptin and should I be getting it?*

A Herceptin is a monoclonal antibody directed against Her2. Her2 is a biomarker that is tested on your initial breast biopsy. You have up to a 20 to 25 percent chance of being Her2 positive. If this is the case, Herceptin can improve the effectiveness of chemotherapy. Not classified as chemotherapy, Herceptin belongs to a new group of treatments called targeted therapy. Her2 activity stimulates breast cancer growth and spread. Herceptin is an antibody designed to target Her2 and shut it down.

The development of Herceptin is a unique achievement. Dr. Dennis Slamon at UCLA discovered the Her2 gene. Drs. Slamon, Mark Pegram, and their team at UCLA were very instrumental in developing the targeted treatment against the gene.

Herceptin is given intravenously either once a week or every 3 weeks using a triple dose. Either method is equally effective and equally safe. Herceptin was initially only used in treating metastatic breast cancer because those were the patients included in the initial clinical trials. The addition of Herceptin to chemotherapy doubled or tripled the response rate and also improved the length of time that chemotherapy was effective.

Two recent important studies support the addition of Herceptin to either preoperative or postoperative chemotherapy programs. In 2004, Dr. Aman Buzdar from M. D. Anderson reported, at the ASCO national meetings, a study using Herceptin with chemotherapy prior to breast surgery. The study was stopped prematurely by the researchers because the patients receiving Herceptin had such superior results. In those patients receiving preoperative chemotherapy and Herceptin, 2 out of every 3 patients had no residual detectable cancer left within the breast by the time that surgery was performed. That was a very remarkable result compared to previous regimens using only preoperative chemotherapy.

A second important study was reported at the ASCO national meetings in 2005 by Dr. Edmond Romond from the University of Kentucky. This was a combined study from two U.S. national study groups involving over 3,000 patients. It tested the effect of adding Herceptin to chemotherapy following surgery, in other words the adjuvant use of Herceptin in patients who were Her2 positive and lymph node positive. Patients who received chemotherapy and Herceptin had their recurrence risk reduced by half, compared to the patients who received only chemotherapy.

These significant study results have led to the approval of Herceptin as part of preoperative and postoperative treatment in patients who have positive lymph nodes. Keep in mind that Herceptin is only effective when Her2 is positive.

There is a downside, a risk with Herceptin. About 5 percent of patients will develop some weakening of the heart muscle (cardiomyopathy) so that monitoring of the heart is needed. Periodic monitoring is performed with either a cardiac echo or a nuclear medicine test called a MUGA scan. Fortunately, if this type of heart problem occurs with Herceptin, it can improve upon discontinuation of the drug.

Q *Who should administer chemotherapy?*

A Chemotherapy should be given in an infusion center with experienced chemotherapy certified nurses. The nurses receive certification through ONS, the Oncology Nursing Society. The nurses should be nearby to observe for and respond to adverse reactions. This is important because on rare occasions, these reactions can be severe. I'm not in favor of patients receiving chemotherapy in a setting where the patient is not directly visible to the nurses at all times.

SHERRY IS SIXTY-FIVE and retiring as a high school teacher. Twelve years earlier, I had treated her with chemotherapy for a locally advanced breast cancer. She had had a right modified radical mastectomy with 25 out of 25 positive nodes, a very high-risk breast cancer. She was hormone receptor negative and received chemotherapy followed by radiation to the mastectomy area.

She's coming to say good-bye before she moves to Indiana and gives me a big hug. Sherry and her husband are moving to help their son and daughter-in-law raise three children. "You know, I can't believe twelve years have gone by so fast. When you first told me that I needed chemotherapy, I never thought I could get through the six months. I remember being so scared. As it turned out, I really wasn't too sick. You probably don't remember but I was able to teach part-time during chemo, and it went by like a blur. Before I knew it, I was finished.

"Then I totally forgot about the cancer except for the couple of weeks before my checkups when I would start worrying about what you might tell me. I was always afraid you'd find something wrong. But the times between checkups also went by like a blur. It's simply amazing how fast time goes. I really didn't want the chemo back then, but you and Joe made me do it.

"Now, I can't believe all the things I've done since then, the places I've been, and the people I've met these past twelve years. I've seen all my kids graduate from college and now I have seven grandkids. I'm really looking forward to the next twelve years."

I'm often asked why I do what I do. This is why.

14

✳

Which Is First,
Surgery, Radiation,
or Chemotherapy?

Q *I've spoken to other women with invasive breast cancer. Most women had surgery first, while others had chemotherapy first. Why the difference?*

A The standard approach is for most patients to have surgery first because most breast cancers are relatively small in size. If the cancer is small compared to the size of your breast and breast conservation is likely, proceed with a lumpectomy and a sentinel node biopsy. In small invasive cancers, I prefer surgery first to allow staging of the lymph nodes, because there is a reasonable chance of avoiding chemotherapy if the lymph nodes are free of cancer. This is especially true if the hormone receptors are positive, which allows adjuvant hormonal therapy to be used as I discussed in chapter 12. In small invasive breast cancers, your chance of lymph node involvement is about 10 to 20 percent. Therefore the odds of avoiding adjuvant chemotherapy are pretty good.

In situations with a large cancer, chemotherapy is often considered as an option prior to surgery as I'll discuss below.

Q *If I'm going to have a mastectomy, is chemotherapy given before or after?*

A There are two situations to consider. If you have a small invasive breast cancer with a large area of DCIS, breast conservation may be difficult from the standpoint of clearing margins. In this situation, a

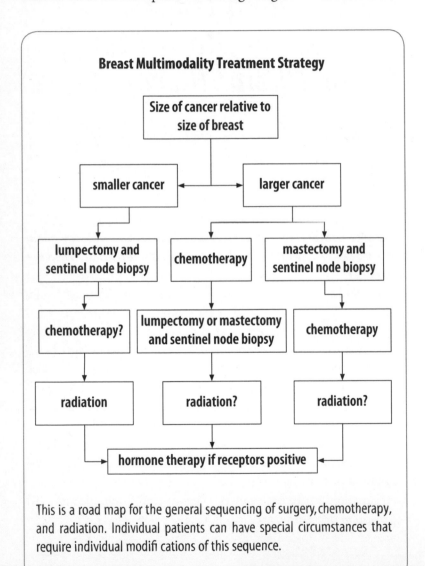

Breast Multimodality Treatment Strategy

Size of cancer relative to size of breast

smaller cancer ← → larger cancer

lumpectomy and sentinel node biopsy

chemotherapy

mastectomy and sentinel node biopsy

chemotherapy?

lumpectomy or mastectomy and sentinel node biopsy

chemotherapy

radiation

radiation?

radiation?

hormone therapy if receptors positive

This is a road map for the general sequencing of surgery, chemotherapy, and radiation. Individual patients can have special circumstances that require individual modifications of this sequence.

mastectomy first is a good option (consider immediate reconstruction, chapter 8). Because the invasive cancer is small, and because DCIS should not go to lymph nodes, the chances are good that the lymph nodes will be free of cancer. This will probably allow you to avoid adjuvant chemotherapy, particularly if your cancer is hormone receptor positive.

The more common situation requiring mastectomy is having a large invasive cancer. Here there is an advantage to considering chemotherapy before surgery. Chemotherapy is likely to be used anyway, to decrease the risk of metastasis. Frequently, the use of preoperative chemotherapy will shrink the cancer sufficiently to permit a lumpectomy.

Q *What type of node biopsy should I have with a mastectomy?*

A If you have an invasive cancer, and the ultrasound of your nodes is negative, and you're having a mastectomy, a sentinel node biopsy (chapter 7) is needed at the same time. You cannot have a sentinel node biopsy performed after a mastectomy because there is no breast tissue into which the node tracking material can be injected. This is the reason that some surgeons perform a sentinel node biopsy with mastectomy for extensive high grade DCIS even though DCIS shouldn't spread into lymph nodes. In performing a mastectomy for high grade DCIS, if it turns out later that some invasive breast cancer is found within the mastectomy specimen, a second surgery to perform a sentinel node biopsy could not be performed because there wouldn't be anywhere to inject the blue dye. Then the only option for lymph node analysis is an axillary dissection.

If you already have a positive lymph node and you need a mastectomy, an axillary dissection should be performed.

Q *I've been told that I have a relatively large invasive breast cancer. What should I do?*

A The first thing is to not panic and keep in mind that with modern breast cancer treatment, you can still do very well even with a large cancer. In large breast cancers, using chemotherapy first has become a very standard approach. Chemotherapy will probably be needed anyway in this situation because of the higher risk of metastasis from a large breast cancer. A breast cancer is considered large if it approaches 5 cm and moderately large cancers are those that are 3 to 4 cm.

In large breast cancers, preoperative chemotherapy has several benefits. Sometimes the cancer shrinks significantly and a lumpectomy may be possible for breast conservation. As I discussed in chapter 7, it's important for the margins of the lumpectomy to be clear to safely permit this. Having a smaller cancer as a result of preoperative chemotherapy will increase your chances of having clear margins.

Additionally, the response to chemotherapy can be directly observed by you and your oncologist. If shrinkage is less than expected, the chemotherapy regimen can be changed. Fortunately, almost one out of three patients treated with preoperative chemotherapy will have no residual cancer within the breast and this is very predictive of a favorable cure rate.

If Her2 is positive and Herceptin is added to the preoperative program, the chance of having no residual cancer at the time of surgery is even higher. So preoperative chemotherapy may prevent a mastectomy and also gives us important predictive information about you. Patients who have no residual cancer in the surgical specimen after chemotherapy seem to do exceptionally well.

Q *Following preoperative chemotherapy, when I have breast surgery, what type of node biopsy is performed?*

A You should have an ultrasound of your armpit before starting preoperative chemotherapy. If an abnormal lymph node is found, a needle biopsy should be done to find out if the node contains cancer. Not all enlarged lymph nodes are due to cancer, as even inflammation from the breast biopsy can cause temporary enlargement, a so-called reactive lymph node. If the biopsy proves that there is lymph node involvement with cancer, when chemotherapy is completed you should have breast surgery with an axillary lymph node dissection (as described in chapter 7). An axillary dissection is needed even if the lymph node disappears with treatment because there may still be microscopic cancer within the nodes.

If the pre-chemotherapy ultrasound shows no abnormal lymph nodes, a sentinel node biopsy can be performed when it is time for surgery.

Q *If I'm receiving preoperative chemotherapy, what are the reasons that I might still need a mastectomy?*

A The most common reason for mastectomy following chemotherapy is the inability to achieve clear margins with the lumpectomy. With chemotherapy, many cancers will shrink into the middle of the mass, like letting air out of a balloon and having it collapse. This allows complete removal of the cancer with lumpectomy. However, some cancers shrink differently so that even though there is a significant reduction in cancer, whatever cancer remains still covers a large area. This type of situation has a Swiss cheese kind of effect with small amounts of cancer interspersed with areas of normal breast tissue. Although there is much less cancer, the overall area containing the cancer is still large. When this second type of shrinkage occurs, lumpectomy will not clear the margins, and mastectomy is required.

You should keep in mind that if lumpectomy is first attempted and the margins are positive (involved with cancer), there is nothing wrong with trying a re-excision to clear margins. If there's still good breast shape, sometimes even a third attempt can be successful.

MARY LOU IS fifty-five, a piano teacher, and the mother of four boys. When I see her for the first time, she has an obvious large cancer of the left breast. Mammogram and ultrasound clearly show the mass and also an abnormal lymph node in the armpit. Both the mass and the node are biopsied and both contain cancer.

I discuss with her two possible options for treatment. Option one is initial mastectomy with axillary dissection, followed by chemotherapy and radiation. Option two is to attempt breast conservation by using chemotherapy first. With option two, the decision on lumpectomy or mastectomy will be made after chemotherapy is completed and will depend on how much the cancer shrinks. With either option, she needs an axillary dissection because she has a known positive node. Most importantly, with either option, she will have the same cure rate.

Either type of breast surgery, mastectomy or lumpectomy (if she eventually qualifies), and the timing of chemotherapy, either before or after surgery, will give her equivalent cure rates.

After much discussion, Mary Lou still can't decide, so I suggest chemotherapy first. Whether she has a mastectomy or a lumpectomy, she still needs chemotherapy because of large tumor size and lymph node involvement.

She takes four months of chemotherapy and I examine her every two weeks with a noticeable shrinkage of her cancer on each visit. After three months of treatment, I no longer feel the cancer and her breast exam is normal. Following her final chemotherapy, she has a repeat mammogram and ultrasound. The cancer can't be detected but she has clips in place that mark where the cancer was located. We schedule surgery, a lumpectomy.

Just before surgery, the mammographer places wires near the clips and her surgeon performs a lumpectomy between the clips. Using a second incision, he performs an axillary dissection.

Several weeks after surgery, I see Mary Lou in the office and review with her the pathology report. "I'm really pleased to tell you that there was only a small amount of cancer within your lumpectomy specimen and there was no residual cancer within lymph nodes. Dr. Jones removed fifteen nodes and they were all negative. The residual cancer in the lumpectomy was 3 mm, about the size of a BB, and the margins were widely cleared."

Both Mary Lou and I are very pleased with these results. She isn't finished with treatment yet and still needs breast radiation and five years of hormonal therapy (she is ER and PR positive). We're off to a great start.

———————————————————— ✳ ————————————————————

Q *If I've had a lumpectomy and I need chemotherapy and radiation, which is first?*

A Chemotherapy should be given first, followed by radiation therapy. This question was answered by researchers at Harvard in a study that compared chemotherapy followed by radiation, against radiation followed by chemotherapy. There was a tendency toward a higher metastatic relapse rate when chemotherapy was delayed. Therefore, chemotherapy is usually given first. When the chemotherapy is CMF, radiation can be given at the same time. Other chemotherapy programs such as FAC, FEC, and AC followed by T (see chapter 13) do not permit radiation during chemotherapy because there's too much inflammation of the skin and deeper breast tissue, resulting in a poorer cosmetic result. When these more aggressive regimens are used, the order of treatment is chemotherapy first, followed by radiation.

Q *What about after mastectomy? Is there a possibility of needing radiation too?*
A There are some patients who require radiation after mastectomy. If you have had a mastectomy, and the cancer is approaching 5 cm in size, or if you have more than 3 lymph nodes with cancer, radiation is given after mastectomy. This will decrease the chances of cancer relapsing within the mastectomy area.

Q *What is the sequencing of treatment for inflammatory breast cancer?*
A The condition known as inflammatory breast cancer occurs when the skin of the breast is red and thickened as a result of blockage by cancer of the lymph system within the breast. In inflammatory breast cancer, chemotherapy is always given first, followed by mastectomy, which is then followed by radiation. Some specialists permit breast conservation in inflammatory breast cancer if the breast becomes entirely normal after chemotherapy, but this is controversial and the standard treatment is mastectomy.

Q *How are chemotherapy and hormonal therapy sequenced?*
A When both chemotherapy and hormonal therapy are to be used in the adjuvant setting, chemotherapy is given first, followed by hormonal therapy. This was not always the practice until recently when a study from the Southwest Oncology Group, a collection of universities and private oncologists in the Southwestern United States, showed that taking chemotherapy and hormonal therapy together seemed to reduce the effectiveness of the chemotherapy. The reason for this may be that chemotherapy has the greatest effect on the fastest growing cells, while hormonal therapy slows the growth rate of breast cancer cells. This may result in protecting some cancer cells from chemotherapy. Protection is not absolute, and patients who in the past received chemotherapy and hormonal therapy at the same time should not be worried. The protective effect was very weak because the detriment of giving both treatments together was small. Just the same, it makes

sense now to give them separately, chemotherapy first, then hormonal therapy.

Q *What about giving hormonal therapy and radiation therapy together?*

A There are no well-established studies that look at this question and most radiation oncologists permit the use of hormonal therapy during radiation. Two studies reported in 2004 seem to indicate no problems with taking Tamoxifen and breast radiation at the same time. Dr. Eleanor Harris from the University of Pennsylvania in Philadelphia and Dr. Lori Pierce from the Southwest Oncology Group reported in separate studies similarly low recurrence rates within the breast and similarly high survival rates regardless of whether Tamoxifen was given during radiation or started after radiation was finished. Neither study was particularly large, so there is still room for disagreement among specialists. If your radiation oncologist prefers that you not take hormonal therapy while on radiation, a delay of six weeks in starting hormonal therapy is safe and will do you no harm.

15

※

How Should My DCIS Be Treated?

Q *How does DCIS differ from invasive breast cancer?*

A As I discussed in chapter 2, ductal carcinoma in situ or DCIS, as it's commonly called, is a noninvasive form of breast cancer. DCIS occurs when cancer cells are present within the duct structures but haven't penetrated through the duct wall into the fatty breast tissue. This absence of invasion influences the treatment approach because the main danger of improperly treated DCIS is the risk of developing an invasive breast cancer. Various studies show a wide range of risk from 14 to 60 percent over ten years. With such a wide range, an estimate of 20 to 30 percent risk of invasive breast cancer over ten years from untreated DCIS is a reasonable approximation based upon more recent selected studies.

Q *How does treatment of DCIS differ from that of invasive breast cancer?*

A If you have DCIS, the focus of therapy is mainly on proper treatment of your breast. The treatment goal is to prevent a recurrence of either DCIS or invasive cancer within the breast. Your risk of having cancer spread is exceedingly low, so that the adjuvant systemic treatments used to prevent metastasis in invasive cancer aren't needed.

Chemotherapy isn't necessary, and when hormonal therapy is used, it's given for the purpose of reducing recurrence within the breast, not to prevent metastasis.

Q *Are there different types of DCIS?*

A DCIS can differ in the size and extent of disease within the breast and also in how it is graded by the pathologist. The usual grading system is based upon how closely the cancer cells resemble normal breast ductal cells. If there is close similarity to normal cells, the DCIS is called low grade. As the similarity between DCIS and normal breast tissue decreases, the grade increases from low grade to intermediate to high grade. The higher the grade, the greater the possibility of having a recurrence within the breast and also the higher the possibility of later developing an invasive breast cancer.

Q *When does DCIS require a mastectomy?*

A Certain situations with DCIS do require a mastectomy. A mastectomy is necessary if the DCIS is large relative to the size of your breast, if the DCIS involves different areas of your breast (multicentric), or in situations in which a lumpectomy is unable to clear margins.

As in surgery for invasive breast cancer, if breast conservation is tried, the margins of the lumpectomy need to be cleared (see chapter 7). As I have mentioned, in DCIS, the required margins are often larger because of the need to have at least one normal duct between the DCIS and the surgical edge of the specimen. This is because in DCIS the cancer cells are only within the duct and not within the remainder of the breast tissue. If the pathologist doesn't see a normal duct between the DCIS and the margin, there is a possibility that the DCIS isn't completely excised.

Q *Can DCIS be treated with breast conservation?*

A Most DCIS can be treated with lumpectomy which is usually followed by radiation therapy. There are certain situations when the DCIS is low-grade, fairly small, and widely excised when sometimes radiation therapy isn't necessary. In the first national trial of treating DCIS with lumpectomy conducted by the NSABP (our national breast cancer study group), all patients underwent initial lumpectomy and then half of the patients also had radiation therapy. Patients receiving radiation had their relapse rate within the breast reduced by half. This study resulted in lumpectomy with radiation becoming the standard therapy for DCIS in the North America. A European study of similar design subsequently confirmed these results.

———————————————— ✳ ————————————————

ANNETTE IS SEVENTY-FIVE and frightened. Although small in stature, she has surprising hand strength when we shake hands. Jake, her husband of fifty-five years, reveals that she's an accomplished sculptor and well known in the local art community. Annette has been getting yearly mammograms since the age of fifty. This time she has a change, a new small area of abnormal appearing calcium deposits in her right breast. Subsequent biopsies reveal intermediate grade DCIS.

"Doctor, I'm really scared. My sister had breast cancer eight years ago and I remember helping her through the mastectomy and the chemotherapy. But she was much younger than I am now."

As I explain to Annette that DCIS is a noninvasive cancer that shouldn't spread and therefore isn't considered life threatening, she begins to relax. "Even though DCIS isn't terribly serious, it still does require proper treatment, because if it's not treated correctly, about 20 to 30 percent of the time it can turn into an invasive breast cancer. What we'll do is have a surgeon remove the DCIS with a lumpectomy. It looks small on mammogram and I expect it to be removed completely. Then we'll talk about whether radiation therapy is needed. It'll depend on the exact size of the DCIS, its characteristics, and how clear the margins are. We don't use chemotherapy for DCIS because DCIS doesn't go anywhere, so you don't need to worry about that."

Annette is now comfortable and smiling. She then startles me as she reaches over, touches my cheek just below my left eye, and presses with her index finger. "Doctor, you have nice bones." I smile back and thank her. I'm pleased that she's happy and I appreciate the compliment.

———————————————— ✳ ————————————————

Ductal Carcinoma In Situ (DCIS)

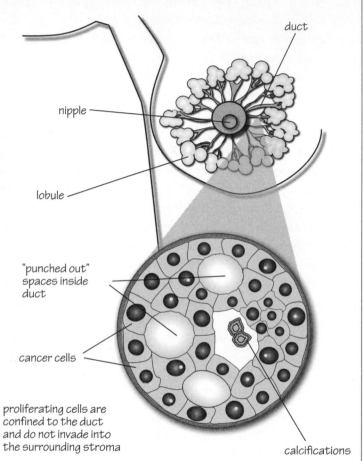

duct

nipple

lobule

"punched out" spaces inside duct

cancer cells

proliferating cells are confined to the duct and do not invade into the surrounding stroma

calcifications

the malignant cells fill the duct, enlarging it and creating "punched out" spaces

Ductal carcinoma in situ (DCIS) starts within a duct. The malignant cells multiply and fill the duct. Sometimes, the duct is filled with a solid proliferation (solid DCIS) while other times the malignant cells form papillary projections (papillary DCIS) or interconnected bridges that surround openings or "punched out" spaces (cribiform DCIS). Some of the holes may contain calcifications or necrosis (debris from dead and dying cells, so-called comedo DCIS).

Q *Does breast conservation in DCIS always require radiation therapy?*

A Some experts advocate treating a smaller low-grade DCIS with lumpectomy without radiation if the DCIS is excised with wide margins, in the belief that the relapse rate within the breast will be very low. This is a point of controversy among experts. Other experts point out that there were no groups of patients within the NSABP trial that didn't have a lower relapse rate within the breast with the addition of radiation, and therefore all DCIS patients should have radiation.

There is a current national trial being conducted by the RTOG (Radiation Therapy Oncology Group) that will omit radiation in some patients with low and intermediate grade DCIS if it is less than 2.5 cm in size and excised with margins of at least 3 mm. These patients will be compared to a second similar group of patients who will receive radiation after lumpectomy. The results of this study will be very informative as to whether there are certain patients with lower grade DCIS that don't need radiation following a wide excision.

Adding input regarding this issue is the NCCN, which is an organization of national cancer centers. Their guidelines permit omission of radiation for low and intermediate grade DCIS that is 0.5 cm or smaller.

In my practice, if I have a patient with low-grade DCIS that is small, less than 0.5 cm, and it has been completely removed with wide margins, I omit radiation therapy. These are usually patients with large breast size, permitting a generous lumpectomy. The recurrence rate will be very low, and with breast cancer screening, there's a good chance that any recurrence can subsequently be treated with another lumpectomy followed by radiation.

Q *Do I need a sentinel node biopsy?*

A The risk of lymph node involvement is very small in DCIS and therefore sentinel node biopsy is usually not recommended. There's significant controversy on the meaning of minute amounts of cancer occasionally found in sentinel node specimens performed for DCIS. Many experts don't feel that those cells have the same propensity to spread to and grow in other areas of the body unlike invasive breast cancer. These experts have raised the possibility that the cancers cells are present in the node because they were dislodged by the biopsy procedure and not because of a biologic tendency to spread and therefore the presence of small amounts of cancer in nodes associated with DCIS shouldn't lead to a course of chemotherapy.

In DCIS that is high grade and larger in size, there is the possibility of having invasive cancer found in the final specimen and some centers perform sentinel biopsy for those situations. Additionally, you should keep in mind that because a biopsy is the removal of only a small sample of the entire abnormality, sometimes a breast biopsy shows only DCIS and areas of invasive cancer are missed. This is a sampling error and fortunately occurs relatively infrequently. More often than not, the core biopsy is representative of the entire specimen.

However, if a mastectomy is needed for DCIS, a sentinel node biopsy should be performed because of the possibility of having a hidden invasive cancer and also because of the inability to perform a sentinel node biopsy after mastectomy, due to absence of breast tissue for dye injection as discussed in chapter 7.

Q *Does DCIS require chemotherapy?*
A Chemotherapy is not needed, because the risk of spread to other areas of the body in DCIS is lower than 2 percent. It's curious that the risk isn't zero and when this occurs it always raises the likelihood of an area of invasive cancer that was not noticed, but nonetheless it's very low and therefore doesn't justify the use of chemotherapy. Because of the potential of significant side effects, chemotherapy shouldn't be used in a situation with very marginal benefit.

Q *Should I take Tamoxifen for DCIS?*
A Tamoxifen can reduce the risk of recurrence of both DCIS and invasive cancer within the breast and also lower the risk of developing a cancer in the opposite breast (see chapter 12). However, there is some controversy regarding the use of Tamoxifen in DCIS. In the United States, a clinical trial by the NSABP showed a lower risk of relapse within the breast with the use of Tamoxifen. However, a similar trial from Great Britain showed no difference. In both studies, the recurrence rate of either DCIS or invasive cancer was low, 15 percent

or less, and therefore the benefit resulting from Tamoxifen would be expected to be fairly small. In the NSABP study, the risk of invasive breast cancer after lumpectomy and radiation for DCIS was between 3 and 4 percent. Therefore the benefit of Tamoxifen in reducing an invasive breast cancer is small because the overall risk is small.

Tamoxifen has infrequent but serious side effects such as blood clots and more common minor side effects such as an increase in hot flashes (postmenopausal symptoms). If you are considering Tamoxifen, your DCIS should be tested for estrogen receptor (see chapter 6) and Tamoxifen should only be given if the ER is positive.

Currently some patients with DCIS choose to take Tamoxifen, while others do not. This is because although the risks from taking Tamoxifen are low so are the risks of having DCIS, making the risk and benefit calculation with treatment equivocal. There is a current ongoing clinical trial to try to clarify the usefulness of Tamoxifen in DCIS, with results expected in several years.

16

---※---

What Are the Main Side Effects of Chemotherapy?

Q *Why does chemotherapy have side effects?*

A Side effects occur with chemotherapy because, unlike targeted therapy, it has some effect on the replication of all cells, not just cancer cells. Because cancer cells grow faster than normal cells, chemotherapy has a much greater effect on the cancer. Still, some normal cells are affected more than others. Not all chemotherapies are the same, and different drugs can have very different individual side effects.

Q *What are the normal cells of the body that are affected the most by chemotherapy?*

A The cells that grow the fastest are the cells within the bone marrow. If you've ever broken a chicken bone in half, bone marrow is the red material in the center. This is where all the blood components are made; red blood cells, white blood cells, and platelets. Most chemotherapy drugs will temporarily stop the production of blood cells and therefore low blood counts are a common side effect of chemotherapy. Secondly, hair follicles, from which hair grows, also have a relatively fast growth rate and hair loss (alopecia) is also a common side effect. The third fastest growing normal tissue in our bodies is the lining of the gastrointestinal tract so that sometimes mouth sores (mucositis) or diarrhea can be a side effect of chemotherapy.

Q *What about nausea and vomiting?*

A These symptoms from chemotherapy are due to the stimulation of receptors in the area of the brain called the chemoreceptor trigger zone. Chemotherapy drugs are perceived by the brain as a potential toxin within the blood stream. This leads to a protective biologic reflex reaction initiated in the brain of nausea and vomiting. It's an attempt by your body to remove whatever is in the stomach, like what happens when you get food poisoning.

Q *Will I have nausea and vomiting with chemotherapy?*

A It depends somewhat on the chemotherapy regimen. Nausea usually starts about three to four hours after chemotherapy and then increases over a couple of hours. It's likely that you will have some nausea that may last for one to two days. With the use of modern antinausea medications, most patients don't have vomiting, or vomit only once or twice.

Q *How can nausea be treated and vomiting prevented?*

A Modern antinausea medications (antiemetics) treat these symptoms very effectively. Over the past decade, the development of effective antinausea medications has been a great breakthrough in easing the illness associated with taking chemotherapy.

There are different classes of antiemetics that work by blocking different neural pathways within the chemoreceptor trigger zone.

One of the oldest antiemetics, Compazine, works by blocking dopamine receptors. Compazine is available by pill and by rectal suppository. The main side effect from Compazine is mild sedation. Muscle spasms can happen on rare occasions and are easily relieved by taking Benedryl, an antihistamine. Rather than a primary treatment of chemotherapy-related nausea, Compazine is now used mainly as a backup for mild nausea that might occur several days after a chemotherapy treatment.

Q *Aren't there newer and more effective antiemetics?*

A The newer antiemetics are very effective and are usually given intravenously, but can also be taken by mouth just prior to the chemotherapy infusion. The newer class of antiemetics called 5HT3 antagonists has reduced dramatically the nausea and vomiting that may occur with chemotherapy. These work by blocking serotonin receptors in the chemoreceptor trigger zone of the brain.

There are currently four 5HT3 drugs available; Zofran, Anzimet, Kytril, and Aloxi. They are all very similar, although Aloxi is longer lasting. They are all very effective in reducing nausea. They also have side effects in common such as headache and constipation that may last for a day. If you do get a headache, you may take Tylenol. If you tend to get migraines, your headache may be more severe and you should let your oncologist know. Constipation is usually relieved by milk of magnesia taken on the day of chemotherapy and the day afterward.

Recently a new type of antiemetic became available. The medication is called Emend. This drug blocks a newly identified receptor called NK1 which seems to be related to delayed nausea and vomiting which sometimes occurs two to three days after chemotherapy treatment. Emend can be combined with one of the 5HT3 drugs if you are having particularly severe and prolonged nausea with your chemotherapy. Emend is taken by mouth daily for three days, starting on the morning of chemotherapy. If you need Emend, prepare to be shocked by the cost, about $300 for three pills.

With the use of these new drugs, chemotherapy-related nausea is usually mild, tolerable, and self-limiting. If you do have nausea with your treatments, remember that it usually lasts only one to two days.

RITA IS SEVENTY-EIGHT and the wife of a retired physician. She's small in stature and appears slightly frail, but she's in very good health and walks a couple of miles every day. She had a modified radical mastectomy for a 3.5 cm cancer with 5 positive nodes. ER and PR are negative, so hormonal therapy isn't an option.

After a thorough discussion with her and with her family regarding the seriousness of her breast cancer as well as a careful review of the potential side effects of the chemotherapy, we decide to try chemotherapy because she has a high-risk breast cancer. We also agree that to make an allowance for her age, we'll only complete the course of treatment if she is tolerating it well.

Ten days after her first treatment, Rita sees me for follow-up and I ask her how she feels. She is smiling and appears well. "Overall, I'm rather surprised and very relieved at how well it all went. As you can imagine, I was very nervous the day of treatment but I ate a light breakfast and drank a glass of juice. Receiving the treatment itself was nothing. I didn't feel a thing. My nurse was really great and put me right at ease.

"When I got home, I was a little tired and ate a light lunch and drank fluids as I was told to. About dinnertime, I felt queasy so I skipped dinner but still drank fluids. I didn't throw up. I still felt a little queasy the next morning so I took a pill. The nausea decreased and I had a light lunch. Other than the nausea, I had a little headache, you told me about that, and it went away with Tylenol. For a few days I felt tired but it didn't keep me from walking. I just walked a little slower. Now I feel all right. I had heard such bad things about chemo that I was expecting the worse. Does it get harder as we go?"

I inform her that the pattern of nausea and fatigue generally remain the same from treatment to treatment without escalating. And based on how well she tolerated the first treatment, I expect her to get through the program in pretty good shape. Of course we'll keep a close eye on her.

Q *What's the main blood problem that I'm likely to get?*

A It's usually a low white blood count (WBC), which results in a small chance of getting a chemotherapy-related infection. You have within your bloodstream white blood cells called neutrophils (also known as granulocytes) that protect your blood from bacterial infections. Neutrophils have a life span of about four hours and therefore need to be made continuously. The infections resulting from a low neutrophil count aren't viruses like colds or flu and you don't catch the infections from others.

If you develop a low WBC and a correspondingly low neutrophil count, you can develop a chemotherapy-related infection. Bacteria that you have on your skin or in your intestines can enter your bloodstream and start growing. This type of infection is called bacteremia, which means bacteria in the blood. Fortunately, most breast cancer chemotherapy regimens have a low risk of this type of infection.

To reduce the bacteremia risk even further, your WBC is checked before each chemotherapy treatment to make sure that it's at a safe level. If you are not feeling well in between treatments, check to see if you are running a fever. If you are, you may have a chemotherapy-related infection and an antibiotic can be prescribed. Your lowest WBC usually occurs seven to ten days after a chemotherapy treatment.

You should keep in mind that this is an infection that you are in essence giving to yourself, not something that you might catch from someone else. That's why we don't generally restrict your activity, because avoiding other people isn't necessary or generally helpful.

Q *What can be done to correct a low WBC?*
A There are medications, growth factors, which stimulate the bone marrow to produce neutrophils. These medications are given by injection under the skin (subcutaneously). Leukine (GM-CSF) and Neupogen (G-CSF) are given daily. Neupogen is used much more frequently than Leukine and seems to be somewhat more effective. More recently, a long-acting form of Neupogen was released called Neulasta. It's much more expensive but one injection can stimulate neutrophil growth for about ten days. So one injection of Neulasta is equal to ten injections of Neupogen.

Not all breast cancer chemotherapy regimens require the use of growth factors. They are very expensive and for some patients cause significant bone pain. There are established guidelines for use. Dose-dense chemotherapy regimens require growth factors, as do elderly patients who generally have lower bone marrow function. Patients who have treatment delays or chemotherapy-related infections due to low white blood cell count also require growth factors.

The growth factors are safe, and usually free of side effects except for discomfort that can occur in the bones as a result of bone marrow stimulation. Mild to moderate pain can occur in various bones in

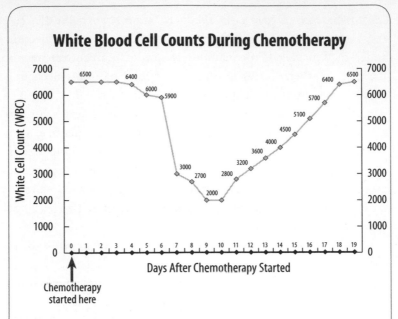

White Blood Cell Counts During Chemotherapy

Days After Chemotherapy Started

Chemotherapy started here

The WBC is lowest 7-10 days following chemotherapy and generally doesn't reach a level that causes significant infection risk. WBC recovery usually occurs after several days and fairly rapidly.

different patients, such as in the skull, shoulders, breast bone, along the spine, and pelvic bones. Usually, if pain occurs it's mild and can be treated with Tylenol or similar medication. The discomfort can last for several days and will diminish on its own.

Q *What is anemia?*

A This is a low red blood count and is usually measured by hemoglobin level or hematocrit. Hemoglobin is the protein in red blood cells that carries oxygen, and is usually one-third the level of the hematocrit, which is the volume of red blood cells present within the blood. The term anemia refers to low levels of hemoglobin or hematocrit and leads to symptoms of tiredness. If the degree of anemia increases, you can also have shortness of breath with activity. Unlike a low neutrophil count, which can develop after one chemotherapy treatment, anemia will usually only occur after several treatments because red blood cells have a life span of 120 days.

Q *Can anemia be treated in a way similar to treatment of a low WBC?*

A Yes, there are also growth factors that can be given by injection under the skin, called Procrit and Aranesp which can correct anemia. These are synthetic forms of erythropoietin, a naturally occurring protein made by the kidneys that stimulates red blood cell production. There are well-established guidelines determining when these medicines should be used because they are also very expensive. They are very effective in correcting anemia and reducing the fatigue from chemotherapy. They have few side effects although there is potential for problems if the red blood count becomes abnormally elevated. Hemoglobin and hematocrit levels need to be monitored with a blood count before each injection.

Both Procrit and Aranesp may take several weeks to begin to raise the hemoglobin and correct the anemia. If anemia is severe and needs quick correction, a blood transfusion with packed red blood cells (PRBC) can be given. The use of blood growth factors has vastly improved the safety of chemotherapy treatments and also has made the quality of life for patients on chemotherapy much better.

Q *What about low platelet counts?*

A Platelets are the component of your blood that stop bleeding by starting a blood clot at any site of injury. Most breast cancer chemotherapy regimens cause only a slight drop in platelet count, with rapid recovery in time for the next treatment. Platelets have a life span of about ten days. Although there is also a growth factor, Neumega, for raising platelet counts, it's rather ineffective and has significant side effects. Therefore, Neumega is only infrequently used.

To correct a very low platelet count, platelet transfusions (a platelet phoresis) can be given. The effect of a platelet transfusion on raising platelet levels is brief, lasting only one to two days.

You're very unlikely to need platelet transfusions while on breast cancer adjuvant chemotherapy. However if platelets decrease a moderate amount, you may be advised to stop taking aspirin and non-steroidal anti-inflammatory drugs because they make your platelets not work as well. This is why aspirin and similar medicines are used to prevent heart attacks and strokes; they prevent blood clots by decreasing platelet function.

Q *How are the all the blood components measured?*

A They're tested in your CBC, your complete blood count. All of the following blood components are available on a CBC; white blood count, hemoglobin/hematocrit, and platelet count. The CBC will also identify the amounts of various components of the white blood count in the part of the test called the differential. You may ask your oncologist for copies of your tests so that you can also monitor these numbers.

Q *When am I going to lose my hair?*

A Hair loss (alopecia) usually occurs starting several weeks after your first chemotherapy treatment. This is always extremely upsetting and it's difficult to prepare for the emotional impact of this. You should keep in mind that the hair loss is temporary and that hair will start to grow back after chemotherapy is finished. I would advise you to purchase a wig; a good wig shop will make excellent and attractive wigs. Many insurance policies will pay for a wig needed for chemotherapy.

You shouldn't try to prevent or reduce hair loss by using a tourniquet around your scalp or an ice cap to reduce blood flow to your scalp during the chemotherapy session. There have been reports of cancer recurring within the scalp from use of techniques that reduce chemotherapy exposure to the scalp.

As your hair grows back, it is usually curlier and darker, and may remain so for several years. Not everyone loses hair with chemotherapy. In particular, the CMF regimen usually does not cause hair loss. If you don't loose your hair, it doesn't mean that the chemotherapy isn't working. It's just that you were lucky and didn't have that particular side effect.

LINDA IS FIFTY-FOUR, single, and works for an insurance company. She's five feet four inches and 155 pounds. I'm seeing her just prior to her third chemotherapy treatment and she seems well. Her appearance is rather striking. Her head is completely bald. She doesn't wear a wig or cap. She has on huge green earrings, large amounts of green eye shadow, and her eyes are bright. I smile, telling her that I like the way she looks.

Linda laughs and shares her story with me. "You know, I was pretty nervous to start with but I felt pretty good after my first chemo. I felt sick for two to three days. I did throw up once but after several days, I felt pretty good. The second chemo was about the same. So I decided to go back to work and I called my boss. He's really great. I've worked for him for seventeen years. He told me that I could come back whenever I felt like it and work as much as I wanted. So I told him I'd try it and see how much I could do.

"I put on my wig and went to the office the Monday after my third chemo. Well, what a big surprise! Everyone in my section, every single person, the other girl, even my boss, had buzzed their heads. I was absolutely floored, to see them like that, and I was speechless. Finally, I took off my wig and just started crying. Everyone had tears in their eyes. I've never felt so supported. Just telling the story is going to make me cry again."

I blink away tears as I listen to her. It impresses me how situations like this bring out the very best in people.

Q *Why does chemotherapy affect my menstrual periods?*

A Many chemotherapy drugs affect the reproductive systems of both men and women. The effect may be temporary or permanent. With breast cancer chemotherapy, there is the chance that your ovaries will be affected and lead to infertility. This becomes more likely with increased age. If this occurs your periods will stop. But as you know, sometimes missed periods happen just because of stress. If you're missing periods and you're also having hot flashes, it's likely that your periods are stopping as a direct result of chemotherapy. You may be going into menopause from the chemotherapy.

You are advised to always use non-hormonal birth control to avoid pregnancy while on treatment. It's very possible for your periods to return after an absence of many months, so care must be taken to prevent unwanted pregnancy.

If you wish to try to maintain the ability to have children, you should discuss this with your oncologist and also with an infertility specialist. There are some very small clinical trials suggesting that use of Depolupron or Zoladex (see chapter 12) while receiving chemotherapy may have a partial protective effect on fertility by stopping ovulation during the four to six months of chemotherapy treatment. Additionally, in special circumstances, I've sometimes altered the chemotherapy regimen to try to reduce the infertility risk. There are significant newer options currently being developed that are likely to be available more routinely in the future, including freezing embryos and egg harvesting.

Q *What is chemo brain?*

A Several years ago, it was reported that some women who completed chemotherapy for breast cancer had noticed some decreased ability to think and concentrate. The women coined the phrase "chemo brain." Studies do seem to support that thinking processes may be adversely affected with chemotherapy for breast cancer.

We recently completed a study with UCLA testing mental ability in women before and after breast chemotherapy. The study indicated that there was some decline in the ability to perform certain mental tasks. Other studies have reported that this problem improves over several years. Although this problem occurs with treatment, its cause may not be directly related to chemotherapy. Thinking problems aren't frequently reported in women receiving chemotherapy for other kinds of cancers, even when the same chemotherapy drugs are used.

What is unique in breast cancer is that menopausal problems are approached very differently. When chemotherapy causes menopause in breast cancer patients, hormone replacement therapy with estrogen is not permitted. Also postmenopausal breast cancer patients on estrogen are instructed to stop taking estrogen immediately, rather than gradually decreasing the dose over many months to avoid hot flashes.

This sudden onset of menopause symptoms usually doesn't occur in other cancer situations. It does happen very routinely in breast cancer patients and they may suffer through many months of severe hot flashes that significantly disrupt sleep every night. Combined with the stress of having newly diagnosed breast cancer, the challenges of undergoing treatment, and then being unable to sleep due to hot flashes month after month, it's really not surprising that concentration is affected.

Therefore, although problems with concentration have been reported following breast cancer chemotherapy, the reasons for this are multiple and complex. The good news is that studies show improvement with time. Postmenopausal symptoms do generally decrease with time. Measures to reduce them are discussed in chapter 18 and may be somewhat helpful. Often the ability to think and concentrate will improve with reduction of these symptoms and a more normal sleeping pattern.

Q *What are the side effects specific to the anthracyclines, Adriamycin and Epirubicin?*

A These drugs are red colored and your urine may be pink for one day after the treatment. It's very important that these two drugs be injected carefully into the vein because if there is leaking from the IV into the skin, severe irritation can occur. Therefore you should notice no sensation of the drug entering your vein. A chemotherapy nurse must be available at all times so that if you have discomfort, the infusion can be checked to make sure that no leakage into your skin (extravasation) is occurring.

Anthracyclines can infrequently cause weakening of the heart muscle (cardiomyopathy). With the amounts given in adjuvant breast cancer treatment, the chance is low, less than 1 to 2 percent, and the effects on your heart can be measured with either a cardiac echo or a nuclear ejection fraction (MUGA scan). Unfortunately heart muscle weakness resulting from either of these two drugs can occur many years after treatment and when it occurs, it's usually permanent.

There is also a rare risk of permanent bone marrow damage that can lead to leukemia associated with chemotherapy regimens containing an anthracycline. This risk may be about 0.5 percent (one-half of one percent).

Q *What are the side effects specific to the taxanes, Taxol, Taxotere, and Abraxane?*

A These drugs usually don't cause much nausea. They are products of the yew tree and have rare allergic reactions associated with them. About

2 to 3 percent of patients receiving Taxol may have severe shortness of breath during the infusion. For this reason medications are taken before treatment (often referred to as premeds) to reduce the chance of this type of reaction.

The premeds include Decadron (dexamethasone), which is a steroid, and two medications with antihistamine activity, Benedryl and Zantac. If you feel chest tightness during the infusion, notify the nurse. The infusion will be stopped and the symptom will go away. Sometimes additional medications are needed if shortness of breath is severe. Patients who have this reaction from a taxane can usually be retreated with the same drug given at a slower rate of infusion. This reaction happens only during the infusion, never when you go home, so you should be safe receiving the treatment in an experienced infusion center. Repeated Taxol treatments can lead to nerve damage (neuropathy) that is usually noticed as numbness and burning in the fingers and toes. This symptom generally improves with time, over six to twelve months. About one-third of patients receiving Taxol report some muscle aches two to three days after treatment (see chapter 17), which are generally mild but sometimes require pain medication.

For Taxotere, shortness of breath during infusion and nerve damage occur much less frequently. Premeds still have to be taken to prevent a rare reaction that is fairly unique to Taxotere, swelling and fluid retention due to inflamed leaky capillaries (small blood vessels). If you are taking Taxotere, it's important to weigh yourself every day. If you suddenly gain weight, you may be retaining fluid. Significant weight gain occurs before noticeable swelling. It's important to catch this problem early, because if noticeable swelling occurs, it will get much worse with continued treatments and it can last for several months even after the Taxotere has been discontinued.

Abraxane is a new taxane released in early 2005. It's basically Taxol but modified using nanotechnology in a way that gives it somewhat more activity against breast cancer with less side effect. Preliminary studies show that many patients don't need premeds when taking Abraxane. There may also be less bone marrow suppression and neuropathy compared to Taxol. It's a very new drug and more studies will be needed before we know in what situations Abraxane will work best, and also what side effects are likely to occur. Right now, Abraxane is only approved for use in metastatic breast cancer. Studies will shortly be underway looking at its use preoperatively (before breast surgery).

Q *What are the side effects specific to Cytoxan?*

A Cytoxan tends to cause less nausea than the anthracycline drugs. It also causes less hair loss. It's eliminated from your body into the urine. If the drug remains inside your bladder in a concentrated way for a long time, it can cause severe and permanent inflammation of the bladder. This can be very uncomfortable.

You can avoid bladder irritation by drinking two quarts of fluid after the Cytoxan infusion is complete and urinating every hour until you go to bed. The fluid I usually recommend is Gatorade-type drinks because they have a good electrolyte balance.

It's important not to overdo fluid intake because taking too much fluid can also make you very ill by lowering sodium levels in your blood. Remember that drinking fluid and urinating frequently only has to be done on each day of your Cytoxan treatment after the infusion, not throughout the week.

Q *What are the side effects specific to Herceptin?*

A If you are Her2 positive, Herceptin, an antibody to Her2, may be used as part of your chemotherapy regimen. Studies showing its effectiveness in an adjuvant chemotherapy regimen have been recently completed and reported. When used with adjuvant chemotherapy in Her2 positive and node positive breast cancer, there is a significant reduction in relapse rate. In metastatic breast cancer, the addition of Herceptin to chemotherapy significantly increases the likelihood of response to chemotherapy and also the duration of response. In essence, the use of Herceptin should be considered whenever chemotherapy is being used if the Her2 test is positive.

Herceptin is very well tolerated with very minimal side effects. There is, however, a 5 percent chance of getting weakness of the heart muscle so that while on treatment with Herceptin you need monitoring either with a cardiac echo or a nuclear ejection fraction. The monitoring usually occurs every three months. Fortunately with Herceptin, if heart muscle weakness occurs, it often improves after several months of stopping the Herceptin. To reduce the chance of heart problems, Herceptin is usually not given together with anthracyclines, which can also adversely affect the heart.

17

※

What Do I Need to Watch Out for While I'm on Chemotherapy Treatment?

Q *How can I lower my chances of getting a chemotherapy-related infection?*

A If you're receiving one of the standard breast cancer adjuvant chemotherapy programs, your chances of getting an infection related to a low blood count are less than 10 percent throughout the course of treatment. If you're receiving a dose-dense treatment (see chapter 13), blood count problems occur more frequently and usually you will be started on Neupogen or Neulasta with your first treatment. You should have your blood counts checked before each chemotherapy treatment to make sure that they are at a safe level.

If you don't feel well in between treatments, you should take your temperature and if you have a fever, notify your oncologist so that an antibiotic can be started. The class of antibiotics usually used for this problem is called quinolones and includes Cipro and Levaquin. These antibiotics come in pill form and are very effective in keeping your blood clean during the brief expected duration of low white blood counts. Hospitalization for intravenous antibiotics can usually be avoided.

Q *Should I stop working and minimize my contact with other people?*

A No, that's not necessary. As mentioned before, chemotherapy-related infections are usually due to low white blood counts, specifically low neutrophil counts, and the infections are usually from bacteria that you already have on your skin or within your intestines. Chemotherapy-related infections due to low white blood counts aren't viruses or colds so that avoiding other people while on breast cancer chemotherapy isn't needed.

This doesn't mean that you won't catch colds as you normally would but this isn't what is meant by a chemotherapy-related infection. To lower your chance of getting a cold, try to wash hands before eating or touching your face to lower the likelihood of the cold viruses entering your nose and throat areas.

Q *What if I do catch a cold?*

A You may treat it in the usual way with over-the-counter cold medicines. Antibiotics are not effective for colds and at present there aren't antiviral drugs for cold viruses. If you catch a cold and subsequently develop bronchitis, then an antibiotic may be needed. Bronchitis is an infection of the larger upper airways in the lung and the usual symptom is persistent coughing of discolored mucous, sometimes with a low-grade fever. If you do get a cold, your chemotherapy program doesn't need to be interrupted unless you are feeling particularly poorly.

Q *Should I eat before my chemotherapy treatment?*

A Yes, you're advised to eat light meals on the day of your treatment and also on the day after treatment just in case. You should drink fluids so that you are not dehydrated. You can tell that you're not dehydrated if you're urinating the usual amount during the day. Dehydration will significantly decrease the amount of urine you make and the urine will be much darker than usual. Eating and drinking typically don't increase your chances of nausea and vomiting.

Q *What if I do have vomiting?*

A Having the sensation of nausea and then vomiting is a miserable experience. Keep in mind that the symptoms are self-limiting and will usually improve within a day. You may take antinausea medications (antiemetics), which you should have available at home. If you feel that you can't take a pill, some of the antiemetics come in a form that can be absorbed under the tongue such as Zofran ODT, or as a rectal suppository such as Compazine. Recently a form of Compazine for under the tongue has become available.

Make sure that you try to drink fluids, because even if you have vomiting, some amount of fluid will still be retained and this will help to prevent dehydration, which would only make you feel worse. This is important particularly if you're receiving Cytoxan because you need to prevent the bladder irritation that can occur from taking that drug.

Q *I received my chemotherapy today. Why do I have a headache?*

A A headache sometimes occurs from the use of the 5HT3 antiemetics, which include Aloxi, Anzimet, Kytril, and Zofran. You probably received one of these drugs by intravenous infusion with the chemotherapy to reduce nausea. A headache is sometimes a side effect of this type of drug because 5HT3 antiemetics have the opposite effects of drugs used to treat migraines, such as Imitrex. You may take Tylenol for the headache and it will typically go away within a day.

Q *I received chemotherapy yesterday and I feel constipated. What can I do?*

A This may be a side effect of the 5HT3 antiemetic. It usually lasts a day or two. You may take milk of magnesia (MOM) at a dose of one to two tablespoons a day until the problem is relieved. On your next chemotherapy, you should take MOM starting on the day of your treatment. If your stools are hard, you are not drinking enough fluid, and a stool softener will help. The least expensive stool softeners are the ones carrying the brand name of the pharmacy. They look like jellybeans. You may safely take one to two pills a day.

Q *Why is my arm sore where I had my intravenous infusion?*

A Soreness of the arm usually comes from irritation of the vein through which the chemotherapy was given. Elevating the arm and initially using an ice pack for ten to fifteen minutes several times a day is helpful. If there is significant redness and swelling, you may also have a superficial infection related to the IV insertion. This doesn't occur often. You should return to the infusion center and have one of the staff examine your hand and arm to see if an antibiotic is needed.

Q *The nurses are having a hard time getting an IV started. What can be done?*

A If you have had an axillary node dissection, you shouldn't have IVs or blood tests performed on the operated arm, to minimize your chances of getting lymphedema, which can lead to permanent swelling of your hand or arm (see chapter 7). An IV access device may be needed if the nurses are having difficulty inserting the IV into your vein.

There are several options for an access device. The simplest device is a PICC (peripherally inserted central venous catheter) line, which is usually placed by a radiologist into your upper arm using ultrasound guidance. This is a plastic catheter that extends from your upper arm and ends just at the entrance to your heart, at the right atrium. Placement of a PICC line is usually not painful and is very much like having an IV started, except that it's in the upper rather than lower arm and an ultrasound is usually used to make the procedure easier.

There are also tunneled catheters that can be placed in your upper chest by a surgeon. Some are soft catheters that extend from the insertion site which require sutures and tape to keep in place and out of your way. Many patients prefer a port, which is an access device that is placed completely under the skin. Ports require a specially shaped needle called a Huber Needle to enter for IV use. I prefer to avoid these catheters if possible because there's a small chance of infection and blood clots associated with them. However, if a catheter is needed, generally you should get the device that your chemotherapy nurses are most familiar with using.

Q *I received a taxane two to three days ago. Why am I'm feeling very tired and why do I ache all over?*

A As part of your premedication for Taxol or Taxotere, you received a steroid called Decadron (dexamethasone). There is a mild withdrawal reaction usually two to three days later and you may feel very tired. For some patients, aching may be related to this as well. I usually suggest taking Tylenol or Advil (your platelet count will be okay this close to the chemotherapy treatment). If this doesn't work and the pain is significant, then a small dose of Decadron taken for two to three days will usually help a lot. You must discuss this with your oncologist or chemotherapy nurse before taking extra Decadron. Some aching from Taxol itself is not uncommon and usually lasts one or two days.

Q *Do I need to be on a special diet while I'm on chemotherapy?*
A Generally not. Because breast cancer chemotherapy has a relatively low risk of prolonged low white blood counts (unlike treatments for acute leukemia), patients are permitted to eat a liberal diet that includes fresh fruits and vegetables. It makes sense to wash uncooked food well and a suggestion of two minutes under running water is reasonable.

You will probably find that many foods taste different than you're used to and this is typical. It's a result of the effect of the chemotherapy on your brain, the chemoreceptor trigger zone (see chapter 16). Your sense of taste will return to normal about four weeks after your last treatment.

If you are having diarrhea caused by chemotherapy, which is uncommon with breast cancer chemotherapy regimens, avoid lactose-containing foods (milk, cheese, ice cream, creamy sauces) as this will make your diarrhea more severe.

Q *Can I drink alcohol?*
A Current breast cancer adjuvant chemotherapy regimens don't have a bad reaction with alcohol. Having one to two drinks from time to time is permitted.

Q *Can I have sex while on chemotherapy?*
A Yes, that is certainly permitted. As a result of fatigue and some worry, you may find that your desire for sex is decreased. You may use a lubricant if needed. If you are premenopausal prior to starting chemotherapy, you must use non-hormonal birth control to prevent pregnancy throughout the entire treatment program. You must take

this precaution whether or not you continue having periods throughout the different treatment phases: chemotherapy, radiation, and hormonal therapy. If you are using condoms and a lubricant, remember that the lubricant needs to be water based.

If you are postmenopausal, sexual intercourse may be uncomfortable due to thinning of the lining of your vagina. This occurs from lack of estrogen. As I'll discuss in chapter 18, many oncologists permit the use of very low amounts of vaginal estrogen, but this is somewhat controversial and you need to discuss this with your oncologist.

Q *May I go to the gym while on chemotherapy?*

A Yes, for the same reason that you can go to work, eat at restaurants, hug friends, and pet your dog. Chemotherapy-related infections are due to low white blood counts and result from bacteria that you already have on or within your body. It's reasonable to try to avoid getting colds, as it will just make you feel worse, but a cold shouldn't be dangerous. Follow common sense guidelines of washing your hands after working out and before eating or touching your face and you will lower your chances of getting a cold. You may be tired while on chemotherapy and if so, you should consider doing a lighter workout, but fatigue will not be harmful to you.

JODY IS THIRTY-EIGHT, the mother of twin eight-year-olds, and married to Andy, a contractor. She's receiving chemotherapy every other week following a lumpectomy for a stage II breast cancer. I'm seeing her after two months of treatment and she seems to be doing fairly well. She's dressed very cheerfully, wearing a shoulder-length blond wig, a bright top revealing her bellybutton, and low-cut pants.

She shares her week with me. "I had my chemo on Monday morning and felt pretty nauseated for the day. By Tuesday afternoon, as usual, it started going away. Thursday night I went out with my girlfriends while Andy watched the twins. Because you told me I could go out and be active, every Thursday night after the Monday chemo, my friends take me dancing because that's when I start to feel better and they do it to cheer me up. Lots of times we dance with ourselves but sometimes with guys. We're not out too late because everyone has to go back to the real world Friday morning. It's funny but I do feel better about everything afterwards, like I'm still normal.

"This weekend I went to the kids' soccer game. It's so much fun watching them run around. On Sunday we had a few friends and their kids over for a barbecue. My friends have been great and always bring the food and do all the work, even cleaning up.

"Last Monday, one week after chemo, I felt really really tired. I remembered to take my temperature. Well, it was 101. A half hour later it was 101.5, so I did what you told me to do and started the antibiotic. I think it's called Cipro. Then I called and came in for a blood count Tuesday and my WBC was low, 1000. I kept taking the antibiotic and felt better the next day and had no more fevers. So, what's my white count today?"

It's now Friday and her WBC is already up to 5500. "Wow, that's fast. Anyway I feel fine and I'm scheduled for treatment again on Monday. Will I still get it?" I tell her that yes, she'll stay on schedule. She replies with a small smile, "Good. Well, not good but you know what I mean. I want to get this over with, and I also get to go dancing again Thursday. I'll let the girls know."

Q *May I have dental work and get my teeth cleaned while on chemotherapy?*

A If you need a routine cleaning, it's probably reasonable to wait until your chemotherapy is finished because small amounts of bacteria may enter your bloodstream during vigorous cleaning. If you need dental work for something that can't be delayed such as a cavity or a gum infection, arrange the dental procedure for one to two days either before or after your chemotherapy treatment when your white blood count will be highest. Remember your lowest white blood count is usually seven to ten days after treatment.

Q *Should I have a Pap smear while I'm on chemotherapy?*

A It's reasonable to wait until several months after treatment is completed to have a Pap evaluation because the chemotherapy and/or steroids given with the chemotherapy can result in mild inflammation or infection within the vagina. This may cause your Pap result to be mildly abnormal, resulting in the need to repeat it in six months. You're probably better off delaying the Pap smear until after the chemotherapy is finished.

Q *What is lymphedema?*
A Lymphedema refers to swelling of the hand and arm as a result of poor lymph drainage. This is a relatively infrequent problem related to axillary lymph node dissection as I discussed in chapter 7. The chance of having lymphedema from a sentinel node biopsy isn't zero but it's very rare. The swelling results from disruption of the lymph drainage caused by removal of many lymph nodes and scarring of the remaining lymph channels within the armpit.

The degree of lymphatic disruption is much greater with an axillary node dissection and fairly minimal with a sentinel node biopsy. Scar tissue that develops as a result of healing from the surgery and from radiation therapy can also contribute to poor lymphatic drainage. The frequency of lymphedema depends on how it is measured. If breast cancer patients are asked if they have any swelling or discomfort of the arm and hand, about 30 percent of patients after axillary dissection will answer yes. However, if the question involves having very significant swelling that interferes with motion or is noticeable to a casual observer, the risk is about 3 to 5 percent after axillary dissection.

Q *How is lymphedema prevented?*
A Prevention of lymphedema is the main reason sentinel node biopsy was developed, which has permitted large numbers of patients to avoid an axillary dissection.

Patients who have had an axillary dissection are advised to avoid injuries that can lead to infection of the hand or arm on the side of the surgery. These measures include not having blood tests, blood pressure measurements, or placement of intravenous devices on that side. When gardening or doing handiwork, wearing a leather glove to prevent splinters and cuts is advised. Cuts should be treated to avoid infection with prompt washing with soap and water and the application of an antibacterial ointment such as Neosporin. These

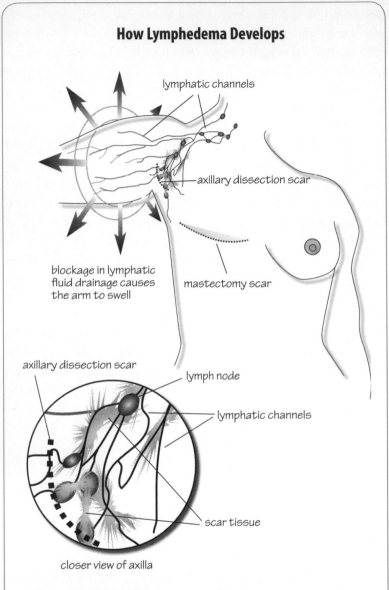

How Lymphedema Develops

lymphatic channels

axillary dissection scar

blockage in lymphatic fluid drainage causes the arm to swell

mastectomy scar

axillary dissection scar

lymph node

lymphatic channels

scar tissue

closer view of axilla

Sometimes, after many lymph nodes are removed from the armpit, scar tissue develops and compresses the lymphatic channels. This blocks the normal drainage of lymphatic fluid from the arm into the blood stream. The lymphatic fluid accumulates in the arm causing it to swell up, a condition called lymphedema.

precautions are life-long because lymphedema can occur many years following surgery.

Some lymphedema specialists recommend avoidance of arm exercise, use of the arm or shoulder for carrying a handbag, use of a Jacuzzi or even a warm bath, and also recommend use of a pressure sleeve for air travel. I don't agree with restricting these types of activities because they don't cause the underlying lymphatic scarring that leads to lymphedema and there are no definitive studies that confirm these activities are harmful. However, these types of activities can increase swelling if swelling is already present from lymphatic blockage. If there isn't blockage, then those types of activity shouldn't cause lymphedema to develop.

Patients that have only had a sentinel lymph nodes biopsy probably don't need to follow precautions because the risk of lymphedema is very low.

Q *How is lymphedema treated?*

A It's much better to prevent lymphedema than to require treatment for it. However, early treatment of mild lymphedema can often prevent worsening. There's a specialized technique performed by certified physical therapists using compressive massage and pressure wrapping of the arm and hand that has some degree of success. For very severe cases, there is a microsurgical technique performed by specialized plastic surgeons to attempt to improve lymph flow through the arm. This is a very difficult surgery and many plastic surgeons are unable to perform it.

18

❋

What Can I Do to Make My Treatments Easier?

Q *How can I prepare myself emotionally for treatment? All of this seems so overwhelming.*

A One important aspect of preparing for treatment is to marshal as much emotional support and outside help as possible. It is very difficult to go through something as hard as cancer treatment all by yourself. I advise you to tell your family members, friends, and co-workers of your situation to permit them to pitch in, to offer help and emotional support.

There is no embarrassment in having breast cancer. Many famous public women including national leaders and actresses are very open about their illness. I consider it a mistake to not tell others and to pretend that nothing is wrong. In twenty years of practice, I've found that informing others is helpful and tends to bring out the very best in people. They will want to help you, and you should let them. Allow co-workers to do some of your tasks at work. Have neighbors and friends prepare some meals, drive or pick up your kids, and walk your dog. Have your husband help with the kids' homework, and with the housework and preparing meals. The kids need to step up their contribution as well. Allow your community to rally around you. The treatments will be mostly completed within six to seven months and it's really not too much to ask. After all, you would do the same for them.

Q *I have young children. Should I tell them?*

A I would advise you to tell them. With this situation, there is no way that you aren't under a lot of stress. You will often be preoccupied, seeming distant, and you'll likely be short-tempered and more emotional. Your kids will sense that something is wrong without you telling them. They may feel responsible for your behavior and think that you disapprove of them or love them less.

This is all unnecessary. Honesty is still the best policy. Tell your kids that you have an illness and tell them what it is, breast cancer. Let them know that the breast cancer will require the treatment of several doctors. Tell them that you're worried about having it and that the treatments may make you feel poorly for a few days at a time. The family routine will be changed but eventually you should be okay and things will get back to normal.

With this kind of openness, both you and your family will cope with this illness much better, both short term and, equally important, over the long term. The kids will understand why things are different. They won't think that the temporary changes in the family life are their fault.

Q *Do young kids need to know anything else?*

A Small children tend to have magical thinking and often feel that they can influence the world around them through thoughts and wishes. It may be that they recall how several months ago while you were yelling at them, they wished that they had a different mom. It's important to let them know that this misfortune is not the result of something that anyone said or thought. This isn't punishment for not being perfect children. Let your children know that there's no blame.

It's also reasonable to tell them that you are worried but also that you are optimistic that you will be well, because in fact the majority of newly diagnosed breast cancer patients are now cured. Both you and your family need to keep this in mind.

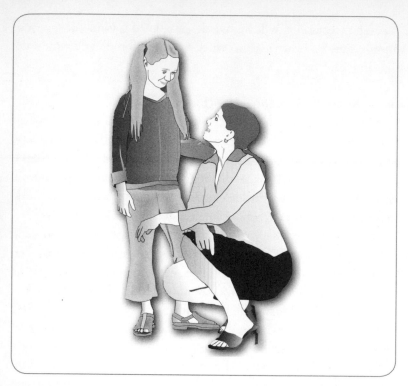

Q *I feel guilty for putting my family through this. Is this a common feeling?*

A Yes, it's normal to feel guilty because life will be different and temporarily stressful for you and your family. However, this isn't something that you've caused to happen to yourself. If you do blame yourself, you need to re-read chapter 1. You are not at fault.

In fact, there may be a very valuable life's lesson in all of this for your children. You will teach your children how to cope with stress, how to live with fear, how to overcome obstacles beyond their immediate control, and how to do something that needs to be done even if it's very hard.

That doesn't mean that you won't have moments when you're sad, tearful, confused, and angry. However, you will carry on. Your kids will see you do this, and when they are confronted with a major problem in their lives, they'll remember your courage and your determination and it will help them get through their adversity also. When their lives hit a rough spot, which is inevitable, they'll remember what you did and they'll know what to do.

Q *Would a support group help me?*

A Yes, it would be of significant help to you and also to your family. Find a support group for newly diagnosed breast cancer patients. Many communities are fortunate in having a Wellness Community that has support groups specifically for newly diagnosed breast cancer patients. Also, a good resource for finding a support group is your local American Cancer Society. There you will meet others who are struggling with many of the same concerns that you have.

Many patients have told me that their illness is always in the back of their mind. It intrudes at the oddest times, while they are preparing dinner, taking a shower, brushing their teeth, or taking out the trash. Suddenly they are overcome with emotion. This is normal.

A support group is very helpful because through the group, you have a safety valve. Instead of continually dealing with your thoughts and emotions about the cancer and the treatments, you can tell yourself that you won't think about it right now because you have a support group meeting in several days and you'll deal with it then.

A number of studies show that breast cancer patients who attend and participate in support groups have an improved quality of life, both during treatment and even years after treatment is finished.

BETH IS SEEING me for a routine follow-up visit. She's fifty-eight and a curator for a museum. More than five years ago, she had a lumpectomy, chemotherapy, and radiation for a stage II breast cancer. She is nearing the completion of five years of hormonal therapy. Her current checkup is fine and as we are about to finish our visit, she says to me, "Oh, by the way, your fan club says hello." I give her a puzzled look so she elaborates, "When I was diagnosed, right after the surgery, I went to the support group. At first, I didn't like it because it seemed depressing to me but you encouraged me to go and I went. After so many sessions, the scheduled group ended because it was only for new breast patients. There were sixteen of us in the group and some of the women felt funny because we weren't going to meet anymore and they suggested that we get together in a month. Well, all sixteen came. So we decided to meet again in another month. And we've been meeting every month since then.

"Of course not everyone can make it every time but most of us show up. I've missed maybe five or six meetings. Quite a few of the women in the group are your patients and at first we'd talk a lot about you and the nurses and of course other patients' doctors as well. Then we'd talk about ourselves, our families, our jobs, and over time we really became friends. Some of the women socialized outside of the group, some didn't, but we'd still all meet every month. Naturally, we lost a few; one moved to Northern California, one stopped coming, and Sandy Johnson relapsed and just recently died. But she still came to the meetings and we all helped her as much as we could. Anyway, because a lot of us are your patients, some of us refer to the group as your fan club and they said to say hello."

Q *I can't decide if I should work during treatment. What should I do?*

A If you enjoy your work, you should work. There obviously will be times when work isn't possible, such as when you are recovering from surgery and for certain days with chemotherapy. Work is definitely possible during radiation treatments. Your treatments won't be made more effective or safer by your closing yourself off from the outside world. Being fatigued won't hurt you or lower your chance of being cured. I would encourage you to be active and participate in life. If you don't like your work, then it's perfectly fine to go on temporary disability. Speak with the benefits person at your place of employment to arrange this. If you want to work, then work as much as you feel you can.

Q *So let me be clear on this. I can lead as normal a life as possible while on chemotherapy?*

A Yes. What most patients are concerned about, because they've heard about it from others, is chemotherapy-related infection. Again, the risk of chemotherapy-related infection with breast cancer adjuvant chemotherapy is low because the interval of having a low white blood count is short compared to chemotherapy for some other types of cancer. The infections of concern are not colds but result from a low white blood count and from bacteria that you carry within your body. Being active and around others should not increase this risk. Eat at restaurants, go to movies, hug people, exercise at the gym, and go to parties. It's all okay.

Q *Should I exercise? Can I make things worse by being tired?*

A If you exercise regularly, you may continue to do so, although there will be days when you can't seem to do as much. If you normally don't exercise, it's probably better to start with a walking program initially, rather than to be overly ambitious. If you're tired, it may be from stress or from a side effect of the chemotherapy. Your blood counts will be checked to make sure that you are not anemic as this can be corrected with Procrit or Aranesp (see chapter 17). Being tired is not bad for you, but use some common sense and don't work or exercise yourself to exhaustion. Be active but don't have unrealistic expectations of what you should be able to do while on treatment.

When your chemotherapy treatment is completed, a regular exercise program is recommended because there is some data indicating that this may be helpful in further lowering risk of relapse.

Q *I think one reason I'm tired is that I can't sleep well. Is there anything I can do for that?*

A This is a common problem. You have more on your mind and it's harder to get a good night's sleep. Also some of the antinausea medicine given with your chemotherapy may make you feel a little hyperactive for that night, specifically if you received Decadron. It's okay to take a sleeping pill and there are a number of them that are short-acting benzodiazepines-like (derivatives of Valium) medications. Ambien is commonly used but there are many others and they may be taken safely over a short period of time. If you don't want to take a prescription sleeping pill, you may take Tylenol PM, which contains an antihistamine to make you feel sleepy.

Q *Hot flashes are keeping me awake and also giving me problems during the day. What can I do for them?*

A You may be having significant hot flashes if you're either postmenopausal and have recently stopped taking estrogen replacement therapy or if you're premenopausal and the chemotherapy is stopping your periods (see chapter 16). A hot flash is the sensation of suddenly becoming very hot and then very cold while getting wet from sweating. These symptoms occur because of lack of estrogen. The hot flashes usually improve over several months as your body adjusts to the lower amount of estrogen in your system. Hot flashes differ in severity and duration from one woman to another but generally gradually improve over several months.

If you're having severe hot flashes, you cannot take estrogen in the form of a pill or patch without a very thorough discussion with your oncologist because of the potential for estrogen to stimulate growth of breast cancer cells. Unfortunately estrogen is the best remedy for severe hot flashes.

Otherwise, the most effective non-estrogen medicines are the type of antidepressants called SSRIs (selective serotonin re-uptake inhibitors) or their dervatives. They work by increasing serotonin levels within the brain, which decreases postmenopausal symptoms. A number of studies show that SSRIs help hot flashes and also can help in treating depression in breast cancer patients.

Q *What about herbal remedies for hot flashes?*

A Many herbal remedies have been touted for treatment of postmenopausal symptoms but most seem fairly ineffective. I'm not sure that herbal supplements that control hot flashes are safer than taking pharmaceutical estrogen. Some supplements contain so-called phytoestrogens, which are substances that have estrogen-like activity derived from plant sources. If the supplement has a dramatic effect on relieving hot flashes, it may be stimulating estrogen receptors within the brain, and therefore may also stimulate estrogen receptors on breast cancer cells. I think that you should be cautious about using herbal remedies for hot flashes because the ingredients are often unclearly stated on the bottles.

Q *Is taking vaginal estrogen permitted?*

A Lack of estrogen after menopause leads to thinning and drying of the lining of the vagina. This may cause discomfort during activity including sex and also can lead to more bladder infections. There is significant controversy with regard to estrogen use of any kind in women who have had breast cancer and you must discuss this with your oncologist and gynecologist. Your oncologist may tell you that it's safer to refrain from any estrogen use.

Many oncologists, myself included, permit the use of low-dose estrogen directly applied into the vagina. I ask my patients to use the lowest amount necessary to control the problem. If vaginal estrogen cream is used, rather than applying a full applicator dose, sometimes just rubbing a small amount around the vaginal opening is enough. If a Vagifem suppository is used, you may insert a dose less frequently than standard application. Another method is to use an Estring, a small ring placed into the vagina every three months that releases a low amount of continuous estrogen to the lining of the vagina. According to Dr. Patricia Ganz at UCLA, all current NSABP trials (our leading national group of breast cancer clinical trials) permit the use of Estring. However, be aware that all estrogen preparations contain warnings on the label regarding use in breast cancer patients.

19

❋

How Do I Know
if I'm Cured?

Q *How do I know if I'm cured?*

A At this time, there isn't a test or a series of tests that can tell you that you are either cancer free or cured of your cancer. Any test that currently exists has some limit on the smallest amount of cancer that it can detect. As I discussed in chapter 9, the blood tests known as tumor markers are inaccurate and can show abnormalities when no cancer is present and can frequently be normal when cancer has spread. Scans such as CT, MRI, and PET are limited by an inability to detect reliably any individual cancer smaller than 1 cm. As with the blood tests, these scans can also show abnormalities that aren't due to cancer. The other problem with routine scanning is that having a normal scan doesn't guarantee that it will remain normal in the foreseeable future.

Unless my patients feel strongly otherwise, I follow ASCO guidelines and don't order routine scans. In medical terminology, there are significant false positives and negatives. A false positive is when a test is abnormal but not because of cancer, and a false negative is a normal test when cancer is present. Therefore it's not possible to determine with breast cancer whether or not you are cured. But it is possible to estimate your cure rate.

Q *How can my cure rate be estimated?*

A Your cure rate can be estimated based on your cancer stage and the treatment that is planned for you. As mentioned in chapter 6, your initial tumor stage usually depends on the size of your cancer and whether or not there's lymph node involvement. The treatments that can cure you include surgery, chemotherapy, hormonal therapy, and radiation.

Depending on your stage of breast cancer, some of the treatments will make very significant improvements in your chance of cure, while other treatments may only increase your cure rate by a small amount. Therefore, not every newly diagnosed breast cancer patient should receive every conceivable treatment possible. In low stage, very small cancers, the potential benefit of a particular treatment may in fact not outweigh treatment related risks, even when the treatment risks are low. When the risk of recurrence is very low, the potential for benefit is quite small.

For example, a 1 cm breast cancer with negative nodes and favorable biomarkers may have an improvement in cure with chemotherapy of only 1 to 2 percent. Is chemotherapy something that you would take for a 1 to 2 percent benefit in cure? That's a difficult question. In surveys of women who don't have breast cancer, the typical answer they give is yes. In actual fact, I've found that after a detailed discussion of the potential short-term and long-term side effects of a chemotherapy program, many women choose not to receive treatment for such a small improvement in cure. In situations with fairly small benefits, I fully support the choice of not taking chemotherapy.

An experienced oncologist should be able to review with you your prognosis and how various treatment options might improve it. Your prognosis will often be presented to you in percentage points of relapse-free survival over a specific number of years because this is how clinical studies report the results. There's also a computer-assisted program created by Dr. Peter Ravdin from the University of Texas,

San Antonio, that can assist your oncologist in estimating potential benefits of adjuvant therapy.

Q *How accurate are these estimates?*

A Estimated cure rates with and without adjuvant therapy are just what they are, only estimates. You are an individual and your future outcome cannot be predicted with anything approaching certainty. These estimates are an approximation of what happens to the average patient with your stage of breast cancer who receives the recommended therapies.

You should keep in mind that it's very likely that estimated cure rates are underestimating your chances of cure for several reasons. First, the pathology staging of breast cancer is much more accurate now than it was fifteen to twenty years ago when much of this data was generated. The pathologists now meticulously go through every removed lymph node looking for the smallest amount of breast cancer including the presence of individual cells. In previous decades, removed lymph nodes would have received a much more cursory review.

As an example, today if you have three positive nodes and the amount of cancer in each node is 1 to 2 mm, it's highly likely that fifteen years ago you would have been diagnosed as node negative. In other words, the studies reported in previous years had patients who were understaged. Their breast cancers were actually more extensive than known at that time. Therefore, stage for stage, you are likely to have a better result than what has been reported in these past studies.

Additionally, the benefits of modern chemotherapy are probably greater than the older clinical trials demonstrated (see chapter 11). This is because many patients in those initial trials received less effective chemotherapy programs and also frequently received less than the prescribed chemotherapy doses. In the 1970s and early 1980s, there was an inability to control side effects and combined with a lack of conviction that the treatments would help, many patients assigned to receive chemotherapy didn't take it. To keep the studies valid, those patients assigned to chemotherapy but not receiving it had to be analyzed within the chemotherapy group. Unfortunately, this is the type of available data that's used to calculate current estimates of chemotherapy effectiveness and that's why the estimates probably underestimate your chances of cure, both with respect to your stage of breast cancer and the effectiveness of adjuvant chemotherapy.

Q *Given what you say about the unreliability of diagnostic tests for metastasis, what type of tests should I have after treatment to monitor my progress?*

A This is a topic that has been studied and debated extensively by experts with subsequent development of national guidelines for breast cancer follow-up. There are a number of guidelines including one by ASCO, our national association for oncologists, and by NCCN, the national organization of cancer centers.

The resulting recommendation, surprising to most patients, is that minimal testing is recommended after treatment has been completed. This is difficult for patients to understand so let me try to summarize the logic. As I have discussed before (see chapter 9), no currently available test can tell you that you are cancer free due to an inability to detect minute amounts of cancer. A normal scan or tumor marker panel today doesn't predict being cancer free in the future because one normal scan today can be followed by an abnormal one in the near future.

It's a well established but unfortunate principle that metastatic breast cancer is not curable with currently available treatments. This distressing fact has been demonstrated time and again from multiple studies performed throughout the world. Similar studies have also shown that overall, finding metastatic cancer earlier rather than later does not help patients live longer. Regardless of the timing, the treatments have the same degree of effectiveness for response and the same ineffectiveness for cure. Any stage IV breast cancer is already beyond the current threshold for curative treatment. It's precisely for this reason that adjuvant therapy (chapter 11) is given, to maximize your cure rate at initial diagnosis rather than waiting for a relapse.

This doesn't mean that CT scans, bone scans, or PET scans should never be done. There just doesn't seem to be value in performing them routinely. It's recommended that these types of tests primarily be performed when indicated based upon a patient's symptoms. If you're not feeling well, if your symptoms are significant and lasting more than two to three weeks, testing should be considered to see if there's a problem. Generally, symptoms that come and go, symptoms that last for only a few days, are unlikely to be related to metastatic breast cancer. New symptoms or problems that persist for more than several weeks require a discussion with your oncologist.

ELLIE IS FORTY, a stay-at-home mother of two. She's with her husband, Bret, a very bright and successful computer designer. They're seeing me for the results of Ellie's liver biopsy. On a recent checkup, she had informed me that for the past couple of months, she hadn't felt quite well. Her energy level was somewhat down, her appetite decreased, and she just felt that something wasn't entirely right.

Her blood work had abnormalities in liver function tests. I ordered a CT scan and it revealed five abnormal spots in the liver and two in the left lung. So I recommended a liver biopsy to confirm metastatic disease.

Ellie and Bret are subdued and seem prepared to receive bad news. She sits on the exam table as I stand in front of her, her husband on one side holding her hand. I let them know that the liver biopsy shows metastatic breast cancer. I feel crushed and I can only imagine how they must feel. After only brief hesitation, Bret asks me what the treatment plan should be. I reply that I'd like to start Ellie on a very mild chemotherapy to try to shrink the cancer, to control it, and to help her feel better. Bret quickly interjects, "But I want you to treat Ellie aggressively. We should have found this sooner."

I watch Ellie's face as I answer, "Do you remember when Ellie had her breast surgery two and a half years ago? I gave her a very aggressive chemotherapy program and this was followed with Tamoxifen. At that time, I didn't know whether or not she was cancer free but I wanted to prevent a recurrence like this. Do you remember what we talked about and why I wanted to use chemotherapy at that time?" Bret and Ellie both nod their heads.

Bret replies quietly, "You told us there wasn't a test that could tell if Ellie was cancer free after the surgery or really at any time. So we had to treat her then because if the cancer ever spread, it couldn't be cured. You also explained that was why we weren't regularly scanning her because I had a good friend who was working on PET scans and I wanted to have her scanned all the time. In fact we had several discussions about getting scans regularly but you didn't feel it was helpful. Maybe we could have caught this a little earlier."

I'm watching Ellie and she hasn't said anything yet so I answer Bret, "That's right. If we had been scanning Ellie regularly, we might have picked this up some months earlier. If we had, unfortunately, the situation and treatment options would have remained exactly the same. We still would be faced with the same unsatisfying choices." Ellie reaches for Bret's hand, looks at me with a steady gaze while saying in a firm voice, "I'm the luckiest person in the world, I really am." Bret seems puzzled and doesn't respond. I watch her intently and I'm not sure what to say so I wait for her to continue.

"I've had the most wonderful forty years. I've still got the greatest husband in the world and two really wonderful kids. I'm really lucky. And I'm going to try my very best." Ellie is calm, forceful, and looks at Bret determinedly as she says this. I'm humbled and inspired by Ellie's deep personal strength. I'm also going to try my very best.

Q *Even if it won't help me, is there anything wrong with having regular scans?*

A There are a couple of potential problems with routine scanning. The first problem has to do with the amount of radiation that your internal organs are exposed to with standard CT and PET/CT scans. Professor David Brenner from Columbia University in New York estimated the dose of radiation to the lung or stomach from a single full body CT scan to be significant enough that a yearly scan for monitoring purposes could actually lead to a small but significant risk of secondary cancer from radiation exposure.

A second potential problem with routine scanning is that the scans can often have abnormalities that aren't cancer but are just normal variations from the average body or areas of scar tissue from previous infection. It's necessary to monitor these abnormalities with more scans and sometimes a biopsy is needed to determine if a cancer is present. This leads to increases in the amount of radiation exposure, opens the door to possible complications from the biopsy procedure, and also causes a lot of anxiety and emotional distress. So there are significant downsides and problems associated with routine regular scans, particularly in cancer situations where there's unclear clinical benefit.

Q *What type of follow-up should I have?*

A You should have routine visits with your oncology team (this may include your primary care physician) at least twice a year for the first five years. These visits should include a careful review of how you are feeling, a physical examination, and basic laboratory tests including blood counts and a general chemistry panel that analyzes liver function, kidney function, and bone activity. You should learn how to perform breast self-examination and examine yourself monthly. Yearly mammograms are needed to monitor for any new breast cancer.

You should also continue regular checkups with your gynecologist and primary care physician because having the breast cancer doesn't give you immunity from having other medical problems.

Q *Is there a period of time after which I can be considered free of breast cancer?*

A Your risk of relapse decreases with time. Unlike some other cancers, however, breast cancer doesn't have a time period beyond which relapse is impossible. Certainly the majority of relapses occur within the first five years, with fewer relapses occurring the second five years. Relapses after ten years are possible but uncommon. There are some breast cancers that grow at an extremely slow rate. These cancers are very well differentiated under the microscope (appearing very non-aggressive) and are typically strongly ER and PR positive. This type of breast cancer can very infrequently recur decades after initial diagnosis and treatment.

It's important to keep in mind that after five years, your recurrence risk is significantly lower and drops further with each passing year.

20

* * *

What Can I Do to Improve My Chances?

Q *What should I do to improve my chance of cure as much as possible?*

A Far and away, the single most important thing that you can do to have the highest possible cure rate is to follow the recommendations of your oncology team regarding the need for surgery, chemotherapy, hormonal therapy, and radiation. Study after study of breast cancer survivors confirm that these are the treatments that have the greatest impact on the disease. As I'll discuss, all other interventions that are lifestyle or dietary in nature, have potential for minor benefit and can play only a very small role in curing you.

If you disagree with treatment recommendations or you feel that the reasoning behind the treatments doesn't make sense, then get a second opinion either from a respected specialist or go to a university breast cancer center.

Some patients seek interventions that don't involve traditional medical care. On occasion, a misguided patient will choose to receive alternative care instead of the standard proven medical treatments shown to cure breast cancer, unfortunately with devastating results. These types of unconventional interventions have been recently given the term complementary and alternative medicine and we will discuss them shortly.

Many patients wish to examine their lifestyle and make beneficial changes to improve their cure rate. If you're considering this, it's very important to understand the difference between factors that may lead to the development of a cancer versus treatments that can cure the cancer. In the case of breast cancer, there are many known risk factors that increase the chance of developing breast cancer, but studies show that changing most of those risk factors after cancer occurs doesn't necessarily lead to meaningful improvement in cure rates.

For example, we all know that smoking causes lung cancer. But there is no scientific evidence to show that after a smoker gets lung cancer, stopping smoking will significantly improve the cure rate. This is sadly demonstrated year after year.

It's very unrealistic to expect that changing your diet and taking supplements would in any way approach the magnitude of the impact of undergoing breast surgery and chemotherapy on your surviving breast cancer. Don't give into wishful thinking. Try to keep things in perspective.

Q *Will changing my diet improve my chances? What if I eliminate meat and fatty foods from my diet?*

A This has been a very difficult topic to study because dietary habits go hand in hand with other lifestyle factors such as body weight and level of exercise. Patients who tend to eat high fat and high calorie diets with low amounts of fruit and vegetables also tend to be overweight and exercise less.

This topic was recently reviewed by Drs. Cheryl Rock and Wendy Demark-Wahnefried at the University of California, San Diego. They studied the relationship between breast cancer survival and high fat diets. Diets that were higher in fat at the time of breast cancer diagnosis seemed to result in a slight decrease in breast cancer survival in five out of twelve studies. Whether this was directly related to high fat diets or to being overweight was unclear, and I'll discuss body weight later in this chapter.

Until 2005, it was hard to show that changing diet after getting breast cancer helped patients live longer. However, all that changed in a landmark study presented by Dr. Rowan Chlebowski (from Harbor-UCLA in Torrance, California) at the ASCO national cancer meetings in the spring of 2005. He reported on the WINS study, the Women's Intervention Nutrition Study, a randomized study of diet in 2,500 new breast cancer patients. About half of the patients were selected to receive counseling sessions to lower dietary fat and were also monitored to see if they could actually stay on the diet. In women receiving dietary counseling and monitoring, the average decrease in dietary fat intake was about 40 percent, compared to the women in whom no specific change in diet was recommended. All other breast cancer treatment remained the same in terms of surgery, radiation, chemotherapy and hormonal therapy. The only thing that was different was the change in diet.

Very gratifyingly, women on the lower fat diet had a significant decrease in breast cancer recurrence at the five-year mark. What is unclear at this time is whether the decrease in recurrence risk is directly related to following a low-fat diet or is the result of weight loss, because the patients on the low-fat diet also lost a significant amount of weight. Several studies have shown that overweight patients consistently seem to have a somewhat worse breast cancer outcome.

The WINS study was limited to women forty-eight years and older, postmenopausal patients, but it's not unreasonable to consider a lower fat diet no matter what your age or menopausal status. There are many other health benefits with low-fat diets, such as weight reduction and lower risks of diabetes, heart disease, and vascular disease.

Reports of two other important diet studies, one in breast cancer patients and another in otherwise healthy women, are anticipated with interest over the next few years. The Women's Healthy Eating and Lifestyle study will evaluate both dietary fat reduction and increased vegetable and fruit intake in new breast cancer patients. In another important study, the Women's Health Initiative Dietary Modification trial will test the effect of lowering fat while increasing vegetable and fruit consumption in postmenopausal women who don't have cancer to see if those lifestyle changes in later life can lower breast cancer risk.

American Cancer Society Guidelines on Diet, Nutrition, and Cancer Prevention

1. **Choose most of the foods you eat from plant sources**
    - ■ Eat five or more servings of fruits and vegetables each day
    - ■ Eat other foods from plant sources such as breads, cereals, grain products, rice, pasta, or beans several times each day

2. **Limit your intake of high fat foods, particularly from animal sources**
    - ■ Choose foods low in fat
    - ■ Limit consumption of meats, especially high-fat meats

3. **Limit consumption or be physically active—achieve and maintain a healthy weight**
    - ■ Be at least moderately active for 30 minutes or more most days of the week
    - ■ Stay within your healthy weight range

4. **Limit alcoholic beverages if you drink at all**

Q *What about fruits and vegetables?*

A This is also an interesting story and there is data to show that eating fruits and vegetables may improve breast cancer survival to a minor degree. In the same review study by Drs. Rock and Demark-Wahnefried, a modest improvement in survival in breast cancer patients on diets high in fruits and vegetables was suggested. Three of the eight studies looking at diets containing more fruits and vegetables showed a small benefit in preventing relapse. Higher amounts of fruits and vegetables resulted in greater benefit. This is certainly a harmless intervention for most people and I routinely encourage my patients to increase the levels of fresh fruit and vegetables in their diet.

It's important to not misinterpret these results to mean that taking a lot of vitamins is helpful. The same UCSD researchers also reported that as of 2002, there was no study that resulted in higher breast cancer survival from taking dietary supplements such as vitamins. Taking vitamins is definitely not the same as eating fresh fruits and vegetables. I recommend to my patients that they follow the current dietary guidelines from the National Institutes of Health, which advise eating at least five servings of fresh fruits or fresh vegetables every day.

Q *It's too difficult to eat five servings of fruits or vegetables a day. Why can't I just take vitamins instead?*

A You can, but it won't do what you want. There's some scientific evidence that eating fruits and vegetables can help you fight breast cancer, but there isn't any established scientific evidence that taking vitamins will. For women who are on average diets and are not malnourished, vitamins don't seem to prevent breast cancer, and they don't seem to improve cure rates either.

As an example, the Nurses' Health Study reported that premenopausal women eating a diet containing fruits and vegetables as opposed to taking vitamin pills had a somewhat lower risk of getting breast cancer. Five servings of fruits and vegetables were better than two servings as reported by Dr. Zhang at Harvard. There was no reduction in breast cancer risk from taking large doses of vitamin C or vitamin E. In this study, the benefit of vitamin A was unclear, but other studies have shown no benefit for vitamin A in cancer prevention.

It's very likely that the benefits of eating broccoli or spinach go beyond the known vitamins that the vegetables contain, and that there's a complex of beneficial factors that haven't yet been successfully replicated in a pill.

Q *Everyone tells me to try a macrobiotic diet. What is that?*

A Macrobiotic diets have well-publicized anecdotes about cancer remission. These diets are usually vegetarian and whole grain. The most radical macrobiotic diet is the one where you are restricted to eating only brown rice. These diets were the subject of review by a team of experts including Dr. David Eisenberg, an expert on unconventional medicine at Harvard. Although the concept of macrobiotic diet in treating cancer has been around in the lay press for well over twenty-five years, as of 2002 there have been no scientific studies evaluating its effectiveness in causing cancer remissions.

In large part this is due to the absolute lack of sound basic science supporting this strategy and also the potential harm that these types of diets can induce. Restricting calories in patients who are often malnourished because of cancer-related metabolic problems is unwise. Many macrobiotic diets are high in phytoestrogens and could be potentially harmful in hormone receptor positive breast cancer patients.

In over twenty years of experience treating cancer patients, I've had numerous patients attempt various macrobiotic diets and I have never seen a single remission induced as a result.

MARGIE IS FIFTY-SEVEN, an interior decorator, and mother of four. Her husband, an advertising consultant, often works out of town. She is one year out from completion of adjuvant chemotherapy for stage II breast cancer. She is seeing me for her routine follow-up and she seems distressed. I ask her why she seems harried and upset.

"Well, for one thing, I'm so busy that I hardly have time to think. But what really bugs me is that I'm constantly bombarded by family and friends with articles and stories about things that I should be doing to stay healthy. I get all sorts of unwanted advice. I should be a vegetarian, I should only eat organic foods, I should stop eating sugar, I should see a holistic doctor to have my body chemistry adjusted, I should take these pills or those pills. Everyone gives me advice. It upsets me because it constantly reminds me of my cancer and it also makes me feel guilty that I'm not doing everything I can to be well."

Margie and I agree that it's impossible for her to follow all this very well intended advice. Not only can't she decide what advice to follow and what to ignore, more importantly, there's no scientific evidence showing that she would be helped by following any of those suggestions. This is a common problem for many cancer survivors.

Therefore, I suggest that she focus her efforts on two lifestyle changes that have some valid scientific evidence of benefit and no harm. First, she will try to maintain optimal body weight to avoid being overweight. Second, she will try to exercise three to four times a week. If she wanted to do more, she could adjust her diet. The data is less clear, but eating five or more servings of fruits and vegetables a day may also help her.

Q *Will drinking alcohol lower my chances of cure?*

A As I've discussed, there are studies that show that alcohol can slightly increase your chances of getting breast cancer, possibly by increasing estrogen levels. This is probably a factor that becomes important over many decades. There are at this time no studies that show that drinking alcohol after getting breast cancer lowers your chances of being cured. Drs. Rock and Demark-Wahnefried have also looked at alcohol intake and survival of breast cancer and the eight studies that evaluated this showed no significant decrease in breast cancer survival from drinking.

As you probably know, there are studies that show that drinking in moderation reduces risk of heart attack and stroke. If you enjoy drinking, it's probably reasonable to have one to two drinks from time to time.

Q *If I'm overweight, will losing weight improve my chances of cure?*

A There are many studies which show that being overweight at the time of diagnosis very minimally decreases survival but again, the reasons for this are multiple and complex. People who are overweight tend to be people who have a high-fat diet, who tend to eat fewer fruits and vegetables, and who are less likely to exercise. Overweight women also have higher levels of circulating estrogens. This may be related to the presence in fat tissue of aromatase, the enzyme that produces estrogen (see chapter 12).

Recently, Candyce Kroenke, ScD, MPH, from Harvard reported on a Nurses' Health Study evaluating 5,000 premenopausal new breast cancer patients and their outcome after twenty-four years based upon their weight at the time of diagnosis and weight gain later in life. Women who were heavier and women who gained weight later in life had somewhat higher risks of recurrence of breast cancer as well as a higher chance of dying from all causes.

There are many other health benefits to not being overweight so I routinely counsel my patients that if they're not overweight, they shouldn't gain weight. If they are overweight, they should try to lose weight. You need to be aware that there is a tendency to gain weight while on chemotherapy because eating can relieve nausea and stress. Keep this in mind as you go through treatment and try to use other methods to relieve nausea and stress.

Q *Will exercise improve my chances?*

A There is evidence that exercise can do just that. Dr. Michelle Holmes from Harvard, in a 2005 report from the Nurses' Health Study, evaluated the effect of exercise in women following the diagnosis and treatment of breast cancer. Almost 3,000 patients were studied. One significant note of hope about the report is that all the groups of patients studied, regardless of level of exercise, had five year survivals higher than 92 percent. Women with higher levels of activity had higher rates of survival from breast cancer. What was significant is that exercising just 3 hours per week was beneficial. More exercise was even better but the benefit seemed to peak at 9 hours. Walking was included as an exercise activity.

So exercise is helpful in improving breast cancer survival, possibly by reducing weight and decreasing estrogen levels. This is one of the few studies regarding exercise and breast cancer survival that evaluates level of physical activity during the years following cancer treatment.

There are many other studies evaluating exercise and the risk of getting breast cancer in otherwise healthy women. These studies all suggest that exercise lowers the risk of ever getting breast cancer. This relationship has been well established by epidemiologists like Dr. Verloop from the Netherlands Cancer Institute, Dr. Ziegler from the National Cancer Institute, and Dr. Bernstein from the Department of Preventive Medicine, University of Southern California. Studies consistently show that women who exercise have a slightly lower chance of getting breast cancer.

This should not be interpreted to mean that breast cancer is prevented by exercise and that mammograms are unnecessary. The risk is just slightly less with exercise. Again, it is difficult to separate exercise from other lifestyle factors such as eating habits, weight loss, and alcohol intake, as many of these factors are linked together.

It seems that exercise and weight reduction, by lowering estrogen levels, may have modest benefit for breast cancer patients and certainly have many other important health benefits. I recommend exercise and maintaining optimum weight to my patients as lifestyle changes for which there is some scientific evidence for improving breast cancer outcome. This is not an extensively studied topic and it is hoped that additional studies will support these positive findings in the near future.

Q *Will going to a support group improve my chances of cure?*

A Several years ago there was a study from Stanford University that suggested that breast cancer patients who attended support groups had improved survival rates. It was suggested that reducing stress possibly improved the immune system and therefore those patients attending a support group had better outcomes. However, more recent subsequent studies at Stanford did not confirm that breast cancer survival was improved by attending support groups. There are other studies like this that also have conflicting results and make interpretation difficult.

It has been argued that there are other reasons than attendance to explain why a breast cancer patient going to a support group may do better than a patient who doesn't participate. Patients who go to a support group may be healthier so that they can attend, whereas patients who are less well cannot. Healthier patients who can attend a support group may also be better able to receive treatments like surgery, radiation, and chemotherapy. Patients not well enough to attend may be less able to complete their treatment.

Whether or not going to a support group will help reduce your chances of relapse is unclear and debated. What is consistently clear is that the quality of life both during treatment and several years afterward has been shown to be better for support group participants. That, in and of itself, is a very good reason for you to attend a breast cancer support group.

Q *What can I do to improve my immune system? Will that improve my cure rate?*

A There's probably nothing wrong with your immune system. You can fight off bacterial infections and viruses just as well as anyone else. The reason your immune system didn't keep your breast cancer from occurring is that it didn't recognize that the cancer shouldn't be there. The cancer comes from the cells making up your breast ducts or lobules and therefore has all the surface markings of your normal cells. It's kind of like a spy in the army who wears the enemy's uniform. It's difficult to recognize the spy. Much of the newer immune research in cancer is attempting to unmask the cancer so that the immune system can recognize that the cancer doesn't belong and eliminate it. There are a number of breast cancer vaccines currently in clinical trials.

Q *What about complementary and alternative medicine?*

A This is the name now used when referring to nontraditional medicine and is sometimes abbreviated CAM. Complementary and alternative treatments typically become popular from one year to the next because of fad and not because of accepted scientific evidence. Some examples include coral chelation therapy, Japanese mushroom supplements, shark cartilage, high dose vitamin C, laetrile from apricot pits, and even coffee enemas. Surveys consistently show that 60 to 90 percent of cancer patients attempt some form of alternative therapy.

The basis of many of these alternative remedies is often a reference to pseudoscience. A single simple cause of cancer is identified and a simple solution is proposed. The answer is always so obvious. Using shark cartilage as an example, the pseudoscience was that sharks don't get cancer because their cartilage contains an angiogenesis inhibitor, a substance that prevents blood vessel growth within the cancer, thereby starving the cancer. But in fact sharks do get cancer. After multiple millions of dollars of shark cartilage pills were ingested, subsequent scientific clinical trials in cancer patients showed no improvement from taking shark cartilage, and the fad disappeared after several years when it became apparent to all that ingesting shark cartilage was an ineffective cancer treatment.

The substitution of complementary and alternative medicine for

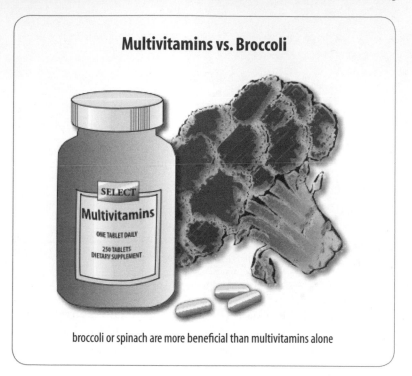

Multivitamins vs. Broccoli

broccoli or spinach are more beneficial than multivitamins alone

standard established cancer treatment can lead to dire consequences. I've seen a number of patients with very curable breast cancer who chose to be treated with only alternative methods, with invariably bad outcomes. They then returned to try to receive standard medical care often after it was too late.

Most alternative medicines are generally well tolerated but occasional severe side effects have been reported. Although laetrile is no longer popular, when it was widely used, some patients developed cyanide poisoning. If you choose to take these types of treatments, you must keep in mind that the substances are unregulated and have not been tested for effectiveness in a scientific manner.

Having said all that, as a matter of fact, a great many of my patients in addition to standard medical care also utilize alternative medicine supplements. I advise them to follow the National Cancer Institute's recommendations that no antioxidant regimen be taken while actively receiving chemotherapy or radiation. In

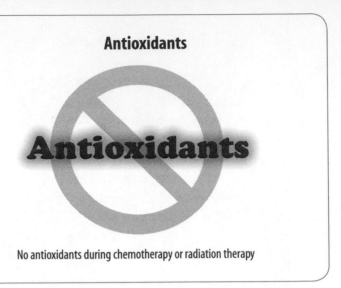

Antioxidants

No antioxidants during chemotherapy or radiation therapy

clinical trials, antioxidant vitamin therapies have been generally disappointingly ineffective. However, the concern is that if a supplement does contain antioxidant effect, it could possibly lead to protection of the cancer. Chemotherapy and radiation result in destruction of cancer by oxidation reactions. When chemotherapy and radiation treatments are completed, then I permit my patients to resume their supplements.

Q *If I choose to take herbal supplements, where can I find more information about them?*

A Dr. Barrie Cassilith is the Chief of Integrative Medicine at Memorial Sloan-Kettering in New York. They have a very informative Web site listed under Integrative Medicine and if you click on "herbs" you will find a list of herbs, botanicals, and similar products that will summarize the ingredients, possible biological activity, possible side effects, and list studies that have evaluated the substances. At this time many herbs and botanicals haven't been sufficiently studied as to effectiveness and toxicities but that is likely to change through the work of programs like Dr. Cassilith's.

Q *If I stop smoking, will I lower my chance of relapse from breast cancer?*

A There's no evidence that suggests that smoking increases breast cancer relapse rates. This answer often surprises people when they hear it. Dr. Valerie Beral from Oxford, England, recently reviewed this topic and found no relationship between smoking and breast cancer. However, there's ample evidence that smoking causes lung cancer, and also, some suggestion that women seem more susceptible than men to the harmful effects of smoking. Some studies show that women need to smoke less than men to have the same high risk of getting lung cancer.

You should know that unlike breast cancer, the vast majority of lung cancer diagnosed in the United States today is incurable. Therefore you should stop smoking, which is something that you already know. If this is difficult for you as it is for many, try the nicotine patches or gum, and discuss this with your physician.

21

---
*

If I Worry and
Feel Depressed,
Is That Bad for Me?

Q *My family and friends are concerned that I have a bad attitude because I'm worried and stressed about the breast cancer. Will this affect my cure rate?*

A You're going through a life-changing experience that has serious consequences for your health and well-being. It's very normal for you to be upset, angry, depressed, and scared at various times. This is okay, and it's part of the expected emotional adjustment that occurs with this illness. Scientific data do not support the idea that stress or emotional outlook affects your chance of cure.

Having breast cancer is emotionally stressful for every woman. Maybe some are better at hiding it than others, but every patient is under significant stress. I don't believe (and there's no scientific support for the view) that a patient can heal herself with her mind, or alternatively, can cause cancer to relapse by worrying. I've personally seen many extremely upset and worried breast cancer patients who were cured, and also patients with incredible optimism who had the misfortune of relapsing. There's simply no scientific proof that a positive outlook improves breast cancer cure rates.

That doesn't mean that having a good attitude isn't helpful. If you have a positive attitude, it makes a difference because the burdens of treatment become more tolerable and your overall quality of life is better. But you shouldn't believe that a bad attitude will negatively impact your chance of cure. That's untrue.

Q *But won't a negative attitude make my immune system not work well?*

A There are some studies that show that emotional state can influence the immune system in very small ways. These studies show minor changes in T-cell numbers, certain lymphocytes active in immune surveillance. These very small changes are of very questionable importance in affecting breast cancer cure. No scientifically valid study shows that mood or attitude influences the cure rate of breast cancer.

As we've discussed before, breast cancer is not one of the cancers for which there's a great deal of interaction with the immune system. Breast cancer patients have immune systems which function normally. The cancer didn't occur because of immune system failure but because of the immune system's inability to recognize that the cancer shouldn't be there. After all, the cancer derives from breast tissue and has on its cell surface, with minor exceptions, all the markings of normal breast tissue.

Q *Does stress cause cancer?*

A That's certainly a common belief among the public. The reality, however, is that there is usually no connection with the onset of breast cancer and the stressful event in question (see chapter 1). With the average growth rate of breast cancer cells, it takes a surprisingly long time for cancer to grow to a detectable size. Many women diagnosed with breast cancer can remember having had a very stressful event within a year or two preceding the diagnosis. As a result of this, they believe that the stressful event such as a divorce, job termination, or a death in the family had something to do with the development of breast cancer. This is simply not true. As we've discussed, the time it takes for a breast cancer to grow from a single cell to a cancer 1 cm in diameter (which is about one billion cells) is about six to eight years for an average breast cancer. Therefore. the cancer was present and growing many years before the stressful event occurred.

Q *Because I've heard that stress can cause cancer to relapse, I'm worried about things that might not go well in my personal life or at my job. If things aren't perfect, will this make my cancer come back?*

A No, there is no evidence for that, either from a basic science standpoint or from accepted clinical studies. I've had many patients with very stressful lives, both personally and professionally, who have had excellent outcomes with their breast cancer.

Q *So worry and stress aren't bad for me?*

A There is no evidence to show that worrying and stress will make your cancer come back. Stop worrying that worrying can have a negative impact on your cancer.

That's not to say that worry and stress are good for you. There can be negative health consequences such as fatigue, depression, decreased appetite, and high blood pressure. So for a better quality of life, it's reasonable to try to limit, within reason, the amount of stress in your life. It certainly makes sense, while you are undergoing treatment, not to volunteer to take on extra duties unnecessarily.

The impact of dealing with your breast cancer may cause you to reflect on some aspects of your life with which you're dissatisfied. As a result of this reflection, you might initiate some changes in your life for the better. You may decide to change your job, to make more time to spend with family and friends, to plan more vacations, to begin an exercise and diet program, to start a hobby that you've always wanted to but never seemed to have the time for, and so on. Many of my patients have taken a bad situation, and used it to initiate many positive changes in their lives.

TRINA WAS THIRTY years old and the mother of one- and four-year-old girls when she was initially diagnosed with bilateral breast cancer. She's warm and open with a compelling personality. Her husband, Rick, is much the same way. You like them both immediately. Trina had previously been treated for Hodgkin's disease when she was seventeen. Physicians now know that radiation therapy for Hodgkin's disease that is given during teenage years increases the risk of breast and other cancers. Both cancers were large. The right cancer was 8 cm and the left cancer was 5 cm. I treated her with an aggressive chemotherapy program and then she underwent bilateral mastectomies.

The right mastectomy revealed the presence of 12 of 16 positive nodes; that's 12 positive lymph nodes persisting after aggressive chemotherapy. Trina, Rick, and our team were all unhappy with the amount of residual cancer in the lymph nodes because this probably indicated a very high chance of recurrence. Trina was very frightened and upset, worrying about herself, about her young girls, and was very emotional.

I sent Trina for a second opinion at UCLA. Following the consultation she reported back to me. "Well, the specialist was very nice and extremely knowledgeable, but as you know, she just had a baby herself. When I started telling her about my situation with the cancer and the kids, I started to cry, and then she started to cry."

Trina and Rick also sought several opinions on their own. However, there was no clear consensus on how to proceed, despite every specialist agreeing that she had a very serious problem.

I therefore sent her for a fourth opinion with the senior oncologist at a famous university breast center in another city. They flew there the night before and returned the next day. I met with them shortly afterward and Trina reported to me what transpired.

"I met first with the resident and then the professor came in. He's an older man, and you were right. He was very nice, very calm, and obviously knew what he was doing. But when I got to the part of my story about the 12 lymph nodes and how much I wanted to live so that I could bring up my girls, I started to cry. And then he became teary eyed and also cried a little."

I looked at Trina with mild disbelief and asked, "Really? And what did the resident do when this happened?" She replied, "The resident had a look of great surprise on her face and then I thought she was going to faint. I must be in really bad shape for all you specialists to be so worried and react like that."

I explained to Trina that although she had a very serious breast cancer, what made the other specialists react the way they did was her wonderfully warm personality, which made the consultants identify with her on a very personal level. Perhaps the specialist at UCLA, because she too was a new mother, saw herself in Trina's place, while the senior professor related to Trina more like a father than as a physician.

I recommended that we give her a second-line chemotherapy program as suggested by the senior professor. She and Rick agreed and she received the chemotherapy and had no problems with the treatment.

I've now seen Trina for many routine follow-ups and heard many stories of how well her girls are growing up. She continues in remission and just started her sixth year after completing chemotherapy. After five years of Tamoxifen, she was switched to Femara.

Even in situations against formidable odds, life can turn out well.

Q *How can I improve how I feel emotionally?*

A It's very normal for you to feel some depression and fear with the diagnosis and treatment of your breast cancer. This is particularly true at the time of initial diagnosis, and, surprisingly, also seems to occur when radiation and chemotherapy are completed. This depression and anxiety when treatment is ending often takes patients by surprise. Much of this is because the completion of treatment is a much-anticipated event and like all much-anticipated events (weddings, birth of a child, etc.), the reality often doesn't live up to what was expected.

Instead of a great celebration and a wonderful sense of relief, your concentration often turns from the constant focus of keeping doctor's appointments, radiation treatments, and chemotherapy infusions, to the sometimes difficult task of putting your life back together. It's normal for this to be emotionally hard because the daily demands of everyday life are routinely stressful. At the same time, you are probably going through a reassessment of your life as well, on both a personal and professional level.

To help you with all this, I strongly encourage you to participate in a breast cancer support group. These are available in most communities and you can find them by contacting the local branch of the American Cancer Society, the Wellness Community, or your local breast center affiliated with your local hospital. Many of the groups offer special instruction in relaxation training, self-hypnosis, yoga, and exercise to relieve stress and to improve how you feel physically. If in your situation, this is not enough, it's perfectly reasonable to have individual mental health counseling and therapy for a period of time until you feel that things are going better. Sometimes antidepressants can be considered, but I've found that they don't work as well as hoped because your depression comes from a temporary difficult situation and not a biochemical problem. Antidepressants tend to work less well for situational depression and are more effective in biochemical depression.

Q *I'm so worried about what may happen next. How can I have perspective on my breast cancer situation so that I can function on a daily basis?*

A It's very important for you to have mental discipline. Don't allow your mind to wander. If you're constantly thinking about the cancer situation and worried about the future, it will definitely interfere with your ability to get through each day in a way that is satisfying and rewarding. You need to focus your life day-to-day, to keep your attention on the moment, and understand that thinking and worrying about the future won't change it.

If you're a newly diagnosed breast cancer patient, remind yourself that today you are fine. The cancer is under control. Symptoms related to treatments will go away in due time and you should expect that your life will get back to a normal routine relatively soon. If you have metastatic breast cancer and you feel fairly well, focus on how well you currently feel, how capable you are today, and enjoy living in the present.

If you find that you can't keep your mind off your illness, you need to set aside a certain part of each day to think about your situation, such as fifteen minutes on your drive home from work, or fifteen minutes during your evening walk before dinner. Then stick to it and when you find yourself drifting into the same thought patterns about your cancer, have the mental discipline to stop and tell yourself that you will think about breast cancer only during the assigned time.

This type of thinking is called compartmentalization and you're essentially putting these thoughts in a box, and opening it for inspection only at certain times. Successful people are able to do this very well, and it enables them to function at a high level even during times of severe personal stress. The support groups are very good at helping patients develop this ability. Focus on living your life day-to-day.

Q *Why do I so often feel afraid while other women with breast cancer in my support group seem so courageous?*

A Whether they admit it or not, everyone is afraid when they have something like breast cancer. Being afraid is considered a very normal reaction. Senator John McCain has discussed the subject of courage, both in his recent book and in his interviews about living with the threat of terrorism. He emphasizes that courage is not the absence of fear, but is instead the ability to carry on despite having fear. Some people are better than others at hiding fear. You should understand that you are demonstrating great courage by continuing your everyday activities and fulfilling as many responsibilities as you can, while at the same time undergoing the treatments that are needed to make you well. By doing all this despite being afraid, you are showing your courage, and more importantly, you are teaching your children and other loved ones how to get through a difficult time in life. Your example will give them courage when they face their own difficult situations. When that time arrives, they'll remember your perseverance, and they'll know what to do.

22

✳

How Is Metastatic Breast Cancer Treated?

Q *What is metastatic breast cancer?*
A Metastatic breast cancer refers to spread of cancer beyond the breast and local lymph nodes. The diagnosis is usually determined by the presence of conclusive abnormalities on scans, although there are times when a biopsy is needed for confirmation. Metastatic breast cancer is never diagnosed when only elevations in tumor markers are present (see chapter 9).

Patients that have positive lymph nodes only in the armpit (axillary nodes) and even above the collarbone (supraclavicular nodes) on the same side as the breast cancer are considered to have localized disease, either stage II or III. They aren't considered to have metastatic disease because these areas are adjacent to the breast. However, if the lymph nodes in the opposite armpit are involved, it is considered metastatic disease.

When breast cancer metastasizes, it typically involves bones, liver, or lungs. The name of a cancer is based upon where it begins. A breast cancer that has spread to the liver is never considered a liver cancer but rather metastatic breast cancer to the liver. This type of terminology can be confusing to many patients.

The majority of patients with metastatic breast cancer have it resulting from relapse of unsuccessfully treated localized breast cancer. It's uncommon for a newly diagnosed breast cancer patient to have metastatic stage IV disease at the time of initial diagnosis.

Q *Why is treating metastatic breast cancer different compared to treating localized breast cancer?*

A Unfortunately, at present, metastatic breast cancer is considered incurable with currently available therapies (see chapter 19). This doesn't mean that will always be the case because medical research is working intensely to find cures for metastatic cancer. However, at this time, it's considered incurable regardless of how much or what type of treatment is given.

This shouldn't be interpreted to mean that not much can be done. Many patients with metastatic breast cancer do very well for a long time. It's just that there's no existing treatment that is capable of eradicating the cancer permanently and preventing disease relapse. This is a very important concept underlying the basis of treatment planning for stage IV breast cancer. The non-curable nature of metastatic breast cancer dictates that its treatment strategy be different than the treatment strategy for localized breast cancer.

Q *What should be the overall strategy for treating metastatic stage IV breast cancer?*

A The general approach is to gain control of the cancer by using therapies to reduce the amount of cancer, while simultaneously limiting the side effects of treatment. This strategy is very different from using adjuvant therapy (see chapter 11) for newly diagnosed localized breast cancer. When using adjuvant therapy, there are specific and limited courses of treatment planned from the beginning. In adjuvant programs, there's an anticipated stopping date for each type of treatment such as 6 months of chemotherapy, 6 weeks of radiation therapy, and 5 years of hormonal therapy.

Conversely, in trying to control metastatic breast cancer, the treatment is open-ended and usually continued for as long as the cancer is controlled. Therefore, many of the treatment choices are also based upon whether the treatment has tolerable side effects over a long period of time. The goal is to select treatments with low side effects that have reasonable activity against breast cancer. In metastatic breast cancer, sometimes a treatment that just stops the disease from worsening, that stabilizes the cancer, is considered successful if the patient is feeling well and side effects are limited.

BETTY IS FROM out of town and was admitted through the emergency room after developing severe back pain during her vacation in Los Angeles. She is sixty-two and she underwent a mastectomy four years ago. She's on Tamoxifen. Her X-rays and scans show small nodules in both lungs and her liver. There's evidence of cancer in her spine that is causing her pain. A biopsy of her liver confirms metastatic breast cancer. I'm seeing her for the first time and her daughter Brooke is at her bedside. Brooke is an artist from New York and for initially unclear reasons, she seems unfriendly.

I review the scan and biopsy reports with them. With the help of mild narcotics, Betty's pain is much less although she isn't pain free. I recommend radiation therapy to stabilize her spine, reduce pain, and prevent further bone damage. Then, when radiation is finished she can return home and see her regular oncologist for chemotherapy. Brooke is upset and completely disagrees with my recommendations. She doesn't believe in traditional medicine and is herself treated by a homeopath.

She speaks emphatically to her mother, "Mom, you don't need radiation or chemo. That stuff is really bad for you. I know a clinic in Florida that can heal you naturally with meditation and diet. I heard about it from some friends. You can be released tomorrow and we'll fly there on Thursday. I'll call and set it up."

Betty looks at me skeptically. I tell her that if she doesn't have radiation, given how her spine looks on the scan, there's a good chance she'll have more bone damage in her back. This could lead to more pain and with time, also the possibility of spinal cord damage.

Brooke glares at me and says angrily, "Well, that's just your opinion. I have a totally different opinion of what Mom needs."

I'm exasperated with Brooke's attitude and I feel that she's not helping the situation. I turn away from her and address Betty with a bemused smile, "Well, there you have it, Mrs. Jones, a total difference of opinion on how your cancer should be treated. What do you think you want to do?"

Betty looks at her daughter and without hesitation, replies, "Honey, you know I really love you very much. But I'm going with what the doctor says."

With radiation therapy, Betty significantly improves. By the end of the treatment sessions, she is able to move about with only the slightest discomfort. Brooke stays with her during the entire course of treatment. She and I actually get along fine the rest of the time. She's very devoted to her mother. On their last visit prior to leaving Los Angeles, Brooke gives me a heartfelt thank-you and we part on friendly terms.

We both wanted the same thing for Betty, for her to get better. We see the world of medicine through very different eyes.

Q *How are the treatments selected?*

A Treatment decisions are based initially on biomarker status (ER, PR, and Her2, see chapter 6) and a determination of the need for rapid response. Some treatments with the lowest level of side effects also begin working the slowest. As is the case in newly diagnosed breast cancer, in metastatic breast cancer the status of the biomarkers is very important, specifically hormone receptors and Her2 status.

Patients who are hormone receptor positive should have an initial attempt at hormonal therapy unless rapid response is needed, because hormonal therapy may take six to eight weeks to begin cancer shrinkage.

In postmenopausal patients, the initial hormonal therapy should be an aromatase inhibitor (Arimidex, Aromasin, or Femara) because a number of recent studies now show that aromatase inhibitors have a higher response rate and longer time of response compared to Tamoxifen. In premenopausal patients or patients on the verge of menopause (perimenopausal), Tamoxifen should be the first choice for hormonal therapy because the estrogen produced by the ovaries will override any effect from an aromatase inhibitor (see chapter 12).

Patients who require a more rapid response to treatment are started on chemotherapy because chemotherapy can often shrink metastatic breast cancer within several weeks. Situations needing a more rapid response than can be expected with hormonal therapy include the following: severe involvement of the lungs in which breathing is impaired, or significant liver involvement with symptoms of severe fatigue and weight loss from decreased appetite. In these types of situations, hormonal therapy isn't a good initial choice because delay in cancer reduction cannot be tolerated. Often patients with initial good responses to chemotherapy are subsequently switched to a hormonal therapy if they're receptor positive.

Q *Why are hormonal therapies the first choice in hormone receptor positive patients?*

A In patients who are both ER and PR positive, the probability of response is relatively high, in the 60 to 80 percent range. Taking an aromatase inhibitor or Tamoxifen has minimal side effects so that patients who are responding have an excellent quality of life. It's important to keep in mind that hormonal therapies in metastatic breast cancer tend to work slowly and initial cancer shrinkage may not be seen for six to eight weeks.

When cancer regression does occur with the use of hormonal therapy, the average time of response lasts one to two years, although some patients can have much longer response times. I've had some fortunate patients respond to one type of hormonal treatment for five or more years. In fact I have a patient who has responded to an older first generation aromatase inhibitor for so long that it has not been manufactured for many years. Her pharmacy fills her prescription by contacting other pharmacies and obtaining the drug from left over existing drug supplies.

Patients who respond to one type of hormonal therapy are more likely to respond to another. Therefore when a hormonal therapy stops working after an initial good response, it's very common to change to a second type of hormonal treatment with a different mechanism of action. Very fortunate patients can therefore go from one hormonal therapy to another (see chapter 12) every few years and avoid the necessity and side effects of chemotherapy.

Q *Are patients who are hormone receptor negative ever treated with hormonal therapy?*

A Sometimes hormonal therapy is attempted in patients who have minimal metastatic disease and little to no symptoms from the disease despite being hormone receptor negative. This is because there is a low false negative rate in testing hormone receptors. In other words between 5 to 10 percent of the time, the test for hormone receptors may incorrectly indicate that they are negative when they are actually positive. Although a 5 to 10 percent chance of response isn't high, if metastatic disease is minimal and there are minimal symptoms, attempting a hormonal therapy is reasonable. If there's no benefit after two months, the hormonal therapy can be stopped and chemotherapy can be started. This is a reasonable treatment strategy to try in patients who feel well and have minimal disease activity, even if they're hormone receptor negative.

Q *What about Herceptin?*

A It's essential to know the status of your Her2 biomarker. This may be positive in up to 20 to 25 percent of breast cancers. Positive Her2 status will permit the use of Herceptin, an antibody targeting Her2 (see chapter 13). Prior to using Herceptin, it's important to confirm that Her2 is positive by using a special testing method called FISH (fluorescence in situ hybridization). This is because clinical trials demonstrate that Herceptin is essentially inactive unless the Her2 is positive by the FISH testing method. Drs. Mark Pegram and Dennis Slamon at UCLA have studied Herceptin extensively. They don't recommend using Herceptin if the Her2 is positive only by IHC (immunohistochemical staining), which is the more commonly used method of testing. IHC is typically the first Her2 test used because it is an easier test to complete and also is less costly. FISH confirmation is important before Herceptin use, because Herceptin is very expensive and it won't work when the FISH test is negative.

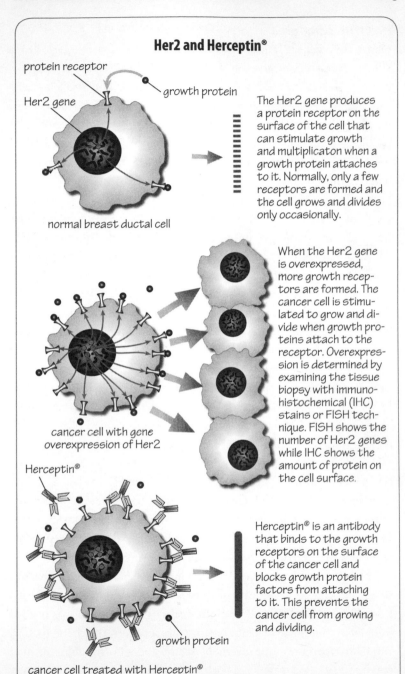

Her2 and Herceptin®

protein receptor

Her2 gene

growth protein

normal breast ductal cell

The Her2 gene produces a protein receptor on the surface of the cell that can stimulate growth and multiplicaton when a growth protein attaches to it. Normally, only a few receptors are formed and the cell grows and divides only occasionally.

cancer cell with gene overexpression of Her2

When the Her2 gene is overexpressed, more growth receptors are formed. The cancer cell is stimulated to grow and divide when growth proteins attach to the receptor. Overexpression is determined by examining the tissue biopsy with immunohistochemical (IHC) stains or FISH technique. FISH shows the number of Her2 genes while IHC shows the amount of protein on the cell surface.

Herceptin®

growth protein

cancer cell treated with Herceptin®

Herceptin® is an antibody that binds to the growth receptors on the surface of the cancer cell and blocks growth protein factors from attaching to it. This prevents the cancer cell from growing and dividing.

Q *How is Herceptin used?*

A Herceptin is generally combined with one to two chemotherapy drugs. When given in combination with chemotherapy, Herceptin significantly increases the likelihood of cancer reduction and also lengthens the time of response. Herceptin usually isn't used with Adriamycin-like drugs because there's a potential of increasing the chance of heart problems when the two are combined. Herceptin does have activity when used alone, but the response rate is lower than when combined with chemotherapy.

A number of very exciting clinical trials are testing Herceptin in combination with a second targeted therapy instead of in combination with chemotherapy. In our practice, through our affiliation with UCLA, Herceptin is combined with either Tarceva, an experimental drug that targets a protein known as EGFR, or Avastin, which is an antibody to an angiogenesis protein known as VEGF. This type of double targeted therapy avoids chemotherapy altogether and is an exciting area of cancer research and gives you an idea of how breast cancer is likely to be treated in the future.

The hope is that these targeted therapies will turn metastatic breast cancer into a chronic illness that can be kept in check for many years by taking medication, similar to what happens with diabetes or high blood pressure. Given these types of advances, it's very important to remain hopeful despite having metastatic disease.

Q *When is chemotherapy used in metastatic disease?*

A Chemotherapy is needed when a more rapid response is required due to the presence of significant symptoms from the cancer or significant cancer in major organs like the lungs or liver. It's also used in patients who have breast cancer that's resistant to hormonal therapy.

When using chemotherapy, regression of cancer and improvement in symptoms can occur within one to two weeks, compared to hormonal therapy which may take six to eight weeks. If chemotherapy is needed initially in a hormone receptor positive breast cancer, the chemotherapy can be stopped once improvement occurs and a hormonal treatment can be started. As is the case with hormonal therapy, there are many different chemotherapy drugs, and fortunate patients will respond to many drugs in succession. This can lead to long survivals with metastatic breast cancer while receiving chemotherapy.

Q *Do some treatments used in metastatic disease differ from those used in early stage breast cancer?*

A There are many more treatments available for metastatic breast cancer than for early stage breast cancer. This is because newer treatments are usually first tested in metastatic disease and therefore almost all new drug approvals are typically approved for use in metastatic disease first. Subsequent trials may then look at the question of whether the approved drug is beneficial in reducing relapses when used earlier in the course of breast cancer, in the so-called adjuvant setting.

There are a number of newer chemotherapies that have significant effectiveness in metastatic breast cancer such as Xeloda, a chemotherapy pill; Gemzar, an infusional chemotherapy with very tolerable side effects; and the newest taxane, Abraxane. Abraxane seems to be very active and may have less side effects compared with other drugs in its class.

A novel treatment of significant importance is Avastin. It's currently not yet approved for use in breast cancer but is likely to be approved for use based on clinical trial results presented at the ASCO 2005 national meetings. Avastin is a targeted therapy that works as an angiogenesis inhibitor. It chokes off the blood supply that cancers need for nourishment and growth. Like Herceptin, it's a monoclonal antibody but it's directed against a protein known as VEGF that is important in new blood vessel formation. Studies now suggest that when Avastin is added to chemotherapy, the chemotherapy works much better and for a longer period of time.

JUDY HAS HAD metastatic breast cancer for seven years. She was initially treated with a number of different hormonal therapies and subsequently has needed chemotherapy for four years. The nurses and staff love Judy. She's a music teacher, her husband an artist. Their two sons are in their early teens. She is very proud that the boys are musicians and members of a well-known boy's choir that requires significant practice and travel.

It's early April and Judy has come to the cancer center for her chemotherapy.

She's dressed as the Easter Bunny with her youngest son dressed as an egg. He's thirteen, nearly six feet tall, and doesn't seem the least bit embarrassed being stuffed into a big white sheet with polka dots that extend from his neck to his feet and filled out with paper towels. Very much like his mother, he's a good sport and seems quite cheerful. They're handing out chocolate eggs to the other patients and the cancer center staff.

Judy takes me aside and gives me a small bag of candy. "Dr. Chan, I want you to know how important the last few years have been for me. It hasn't always been easy, but I've had the chance to raise my boys. Now when I look at them, I can see the men that they will become and I'm so very pleased and grateful."

Q *When chemotherapy is working in metastatic cancer, can it be stopped and restarted, or does it need to continue indefinitely?*

A A number of studies have addressed this important question. Somewhat surprisingly, patients who remain on a chemotherapy that is successfully controlling metastatic breast cancer actually have a better quality of life than patients who stop chemotherapy and then later have it restarted when the cancer again becomes active. It seems that usually the symptoms of having progressing cancer outweigh the side effects of chemotherapy.

Q *What are bisphosphonates?*

A These are drugs that act to make the bones stronger. The intravenous bisphosphonates are Zometa (zoledronate) and Aredia (pamidronate) and they are very powerful intravenous forms of the pills (like Fosamax) that postmenopausal women take for osteoporosis. These drugs are given every three to four weeks intravenously and are used when cancer has spread into the bones.

Breast cancer patients with bone metastasis and regular intravenous bisphosphonate treatments have diminished pain and a lower chance of bone related problems such as fractures or the need to receive radiation therapy to relieve bone pain. The drugs work by reducing the cancer's ability to destroy normal bone and by making existing bone stronger. These drugs are not considered chemotherapy.

They have a few side effects of note. Some patients have discomfort in the bones for one to two days after treatment. The discomfort is usually mild but rarely can be moderately severe and prevent continuation of the treatments. Monitoring of kidney function by blood test is needed as some patients may have impairment in kidney function requiring discontinuation of treatments. This side effect usually will correct itself when the drug is stopped. An uncommon but significant side effect only recently reported is that Zometa and Aredia can sometimes prevent bone healing if major dental work affecting the bone surrounding the tooth is performed. When this occurs, it may be painful until healing is complete. The treatments should be stopped and not restarted until the bone is completely healed. I caution my patients to avoid dental work involving the bones such as a root canal or tooth extraction, if possible, until they have been off the infusions for more than a month and to delay restarting the infusions for at least two months.

Q *When is radiation therapy used in metastatic breast cancer?*

A In metastatic breast cancer, radiation therapy is limited by an inability to treat large areas of the body because of adverse side effects. Radiation is very useful if there are isolated areas that can be targeted by the treatment beam. For example, if metastatic breast cancer is causing low back pain because the spine is involved, radiation is beneficial in reducing the cancer and diminishing pain. Recent developments in radiation technique such as IMRT and stereotatic radiosurgery allow more precise targeting of cancer areas while limiting exposure to normal tissues. These newer techniques allow more radiation to be given to more areas with lesser side effects.

Q *What about bone marrow transplant for metastatic breast cancer?*

A Bone marrow transplant has been shown to be unhelpful in metastatic breast cancer in a number of rigorous scientifically conducted clinical studies. The potential benefit from transplant shown in initial phase 2 studies was not confirmed in the phase 3 studies performed in North America and Europe. The fact that these studies didn't show benefit took many experts by surprise. There was a time when many patients with metastatic breast cancer were undergoing transplant in hope of cure based on the results of phase 2 clinical trials. Many insurance companies were taken to court to pay for this very expensive treatment. When the phase 3 studies demonstrated no benefit to transplant, the breast cancer community was stunned. The absolute importance of phase 3 trials in proving the effectiveness of any treatment will be discussed in chapter 23.

For breast cancer treatment, the procedure involves removing a patient's own bone marrow for freezing and storing, then giving the patient very high doses of chemotherapy to try to eradicate the metastatic breast cancer, and then re-infusing the bone marrow back to the patient to normalize the blood counts. The term bone marrow transplant in this setting is a misnomer because a donor bone marrow isn't used in this procedure. The procedure is more appropriately called high dose chemotherapy with stem cell rescue. It permits otherwise lethal doses of chemotherapy or radiation to be given because the removed bone marrow has been protected from the high dose treatment.

Unfortunately, the results of much anticipated clinical trials from Europe and the United States demonstrated no improvement in survival in comparison to standard chemotherapy, despite the early promising results and tremendous publicity regarding this procedure. In addition, there was a higher than expected level of toxicity and treatment-related death. Presently, high-dose chemotherapy and bone marrow transplant for breast cancer are no longer being performed except under special research programs that are trying to improve the technique.

Q *So metastatic breast cancer is a serious problem, but it's not hopeless?*

A It's very important to remain hopeful when having metastatic breast cancer. There are many treatment options. Some patients are very lucky and respond to one treatment after another with minimal side effects and many years of good quality of life. Breast cancer research receives the highest funding among all the different types of cancers and there's always the possibility of a breakthrough drug on the near horizon.

I remember, not that long ago, when some of my patients who had exhausted all hormonal and chemotherapy options were among the first patients to receive Herceptin in the first UCLA Herceptin clinical trial. These patients had extensive disease and a very limited life expectancy. I think to the surprise of a lot of people (and I must include myself), dramatic responses occurred and for some patients lasted years. Do breakthroughs in treatment like this happen every year? No. But can they happen? Yes, they definitely can.

23

✸

What Are Clinical Trials?

Q *What are clinical trials?*

A Clinical trials are medical experiments conducted with the intent of generating an answer to a specific question. In cancer treatment, the clinical trial often involves testing a drug to assess effectiveness and tolerability. However, virtually anything can be tested for how it may affect cancer treatment, survival outcome, quality of life, etc.

An important thing to keep in mind about clinical trials is that you always have the freedom to participate or not. You should never feel coerced into being a part of a trial.

Q *Would it help me to be a part of a clinical trial?*

A That's often difficult to know for sure. As in everything in life, there are some excellent clinical trials and there are some poorly designed ones. It's very important for you to understand before you enroll, what the purpose of the study is and how your treatment in the study may be different from the current standard of care. Many clinical trials are worthwhile to the participants because they may be permitted to receive a promising treatment that is otherwise unavailable to them.

One example would be the first patients who received Herceptin, the antibody targeting Her2. This was a drug that had a very strong scientific basis for development, was promising in the laboratory and also in animals, and needed to be tested in humans. At one time, the only way you could have received this drug was by participating in a clinical trial. Those initial Herceptin trials were used to assess effectiveness and treatment-related side effects, which ultimately led to FDA approval.

Other trials won't necessarily benefit the participant, but may benefit future patients by expanding our knowledge about a particular concept. A good example is one that we recently completed with Dr. Richard Pietras at UCLA regarding the effects of adjuvant treatment on cognition (a chemo brain study). If you had enrolled in this study, you would have taken tests that measured how you thought, both before and after treatment, to see how the treatment affected your thought processes. This study would not have affected your treatment in any way, but your participation would have advanced the knowledge regarding a very important issue for breast cancer patients undergoing adjuvant chemotherapy and hormonal therapy.

Q *Can I be hurt as part of a clinical trial?*

A Clinical trials are tightly regulated in the United States. Much of the regulation came as a result of injuries that did occur from improper clinical trials conducted in the 1950s and 1960s. Clinical trials today require informed consent. You can't be part of any trial without your knowledge and formal acceptance. All trials are reviewed by panels of professional and lay people to insure that there is a valid clinical question to be answered and that there are appropriate safeguards in place for participants.

You should be aware that clinical trials do have risks. An experimental drug that has not been used by many patients may have unanticipated, rare and/or severe side effects. Therefore, you should have a good reason for enrolling in an experimental drug trial. It should offer the potential for greater benefit compared to standard treatments currently available to you.

Q *What is a phase 1 clinical trial?*

A A phase 1 drug trial is a trial that is being conducted mainly to assess safety of a new drug. You're probably unaware that there are thousands of new compounds tested yearly for effect against cancer. Only the most effective drugs in the laboratory are selected for study in animals. The animal studies evaluate the ability of the novel drug to kill cancer without harming the animal. Only if the drug shows significant activity and safety in animals does human testing begin. The initial human testing of any drug involves phase 1 clinical trials.

If you enroll in a phase 1 test, you are likely to be among the first humans to be receiving the drug. Usually small groups of patients are given the drug at escalating doses. The main function of a phase 1 trial is to assess toxicity or side effects. Only secondarily is anti-cancer effect noted. If the drug can be given safely and some patients also show cancer regression, the drug then goes on to phase 2 testing.

Q *Is it helpful for me to enroll in a phase 1 trial?*

A Phase 1 trials are usually limited to situations in which the cancer is metastasized and currently available standard treatments have not been helpful. This is to protect you from enrolling if there is established available treatment that is known to have activity against your cancer. The likelihood of benefit from enrolling in a phase 1 trial is low. A recent analysis by the National Cancer Institute puts the benefit at 1 to 2 percent. It's extremely difficult to develop effective cancer therapy. Many drugs showing promise in the laboratory and in animals fail to work in humans. For this reason, I tend to discourage my patients from enrolling into phase 1 trials unless there is a drug of particular scientific pedigree with reports of exceptional activity in pre-human testing. I do believe that phase 1 trials are very important for the advancement of knowledge in cancer treatment, so if you are out of good options and you want to try something novel, you should consider enrolling. However, keep in mind and understand that the likelihood of benefit is relatively low.

Q *What is a phase 2 clinical trial?*

A Phase 2 drug trials are studies performed after there is significant data about side effects in humans, after correct dosing has been established, and when some activity against specific cancers is suggested. The main purpose of a phase 2 trial is to see how well a new drug works against cancer. There are many phase 2 trials available throughout the country, usually at university cancer centers, but each year there are only a few very promising phase 2 trials in breast cancer. These are drugs with sound scientific basis for development that have already demonstrated activity against cancer in phase 1 studies. The only way that you can receive this potentially breakthrough type of drug is on clinical trial, because the drug isn't yet approved by the FDA.

Q *Should I enroll in a phase 2 trial?*

A It depends on the trial. You need to find out as much as you can about the drug. How is the drug thought to work? What are the expected side effects? Did patients demonstrate meaningful regression of cancer in phase 1 trials? If you don't enroll, what would your standard treatment be? What would be the expectations for remission of cancer with standard treatment?

A potential blockbuster drug will almost always only be made available in a phase 2 trial that is sponsored through a university-based research group. Competition to get these types of clinical trials is rigorous and the pharmaceutical company will usually want nationally recognized specialists and research teams to lead the study. A good example of this type of research group is the UCLA/TORI research network. TORI stands for Translational Oncology Research Institute. In a program like this, every trial is initially reviewed by the UCLA Division of Hematology/Oncology and only the best trials are considered for enrollment in a network of highly selected community-based oncologists who work directly with the UCLA researchers.

Q *What is a phase 3 clinical trial?*

A A phase 3 trial is the most scientifically rigorous type of trial. This is the kind of trial that is usually reserved for a drug that demonstrated significant activity against cancer in phase 2 trials, for the purpose of obtaining approval by the FDA (Food and Drug Administration). Without FDA approval, no pharmaceutically manufactured drug can be prescribed in the United States.

Phase 3 trials are randomized, prospective, and often double blinded. The term randomized means that a computer selects whether or not you get a standard treatment or the drug being studied. Another common strategy of phase 3 testing of a new cancer drug involves giving every patient the best available standard treatment and then having a computer select a portion of patients to receive the study drug in addition to the best available standard treatment. Prospective means that the study begins at the moment that the treatment starts. Patients are not treated and then later enrolled only if they do well. This gives a much more accurate assessment of what happens to the average patient receiving this treatment. Double blind means that neither you nor your treating oncologist and nurses know whether the computer selected you to receive the experimental treatment or not. This is the only way that a treatment can be scientifically proven to be helpful or harmful because it removes any influence by the researchers on the final result.

It's very difficult for an experimental cancer treatment to pass a phase 3 trial, and success almost always assures FDA approval. In order for a phase 3 trial to be approved for enrollment, experts in the field must make certain that based upon current knowledge, all patients enrolled in the trial will receive treatments thought to be equal to the current best treatment. No patient on a phase 3 trial can receive a treatment which is knowingly inferior. I encourage my patients to enroll in phase 3 trials because they usually involve the best standard treatments available. If you enroll and you are not selected by computer to get the experimental drug, you should at the very least be receiving the current best available treatment for your stage of breast cancer.

Q *So what should I do before I enroll in a clinical trial?*

A You need to do some homework and first read the consent form carefully. What is the purpose of the study? Has the study drug shown significant anti-cancer activity? Are there any significant side effects?

Do the significant side effects occur frequently or very rarely? Why is your oncologist involved in this study? If you don't enroll in the study, what treatment is planned and what is the expected outcome with that treatment? How strongly does your oncologist feel that this study is a good one for your particular situation? Is the study part of a university research trial?

Most importantly, if you have doubts, understand that you don't have to enroll. Keep in mind that you can always get a second opinion and review the option with an oncologist who isn't involved in the trial. If you are still unsure, be comfortable saying no. Whether or not you enroll in the clinical trial shouldn't affect your relationship with your physician.

MARCIE HAS METASTATIC breast cancer. She's an instructor at a nursing school and her husband, Derrick, is a dentist. Marcie has mainly relapsed in her bones, including several ribs and a few spots along her spine. Her discomfort is mild and she continues to work. I recommend that she be treated with hormonal therapy, an aromatase inhibitor. That would be the standard initial treatment for her situation. I also review with her and Derrick an option to enroll in a clinical trial evaluating the addition of a targeted therapy to an aromatase inhibitor. I explain that it's a phase 3 trial. She would definitely receive the aromatase inhibitor, but neither she nor I would know if she was taking the experimental targeted treatment. All patients in the study would receive the aromatase inhibitor. Half of the patients would get the experimental targeted therapy in pill form while the other half would receive an inert sugar pill that looked exactly the same.

Marcie and Derrick ask a number of questions over several visits before deciding. Then Marcie agrees to the clinical trial. "The way I see it, the experimental treatment doesn't seem to have many side effects and some patients with breast cancer have already been helped by it. In the best-case scenario, I'll get the new drug and it may help me. At the very least, if I end up taking the placebo, I'll still be getting the aromatase inhibitor that you would have recommended anyway. So I may be helping myself, but I'll also be helping others. I'd like to do it."

---※---

Afterword

Iғ ʏᴏᴜ ᴀʀᴇ a newly diagnosed breast cancer patient, you have every reason for hope and optimism. If the cancer is limited to your breast and lymph nodes, there is a very good chance for cure. If the cancer is metastasized, there are many options for treatment to reduce your cancer and it's possible to control it for many years.

Find out who are the best specialists in your area. You generally don't do this by asking friends and relatives but rather by asking other physicians. There's a saying that I think is usually true, that only the good doctors know who the good doctors are. Start by asking your family physician, your gynecologist, and your mammographer. Don't be hesitant to see several doctors until you decide upon the ones to place your trust in. If you don't understand the recommendations made or you disagree with them, get a second opinion from a university affiliated breast center or from another specialist. A good physician will never be offended by a request for a second opinion.

When you have cancer, you're bombarded with information from well-intended friends and loved ones. Some of the information will be helpful. However, much of it may be wrong. Use common sense and a healthy dose of skepticism in reviewing suggested alternative treatments. The most important interventions to help you survive breast cancer are the standard ones; surgery, radiation therapy, chemotherapy, and hormonal therapy. Although diet, supplements, and lifestyle factors may play a part in your recovery, they won't substitute for proper treatment, so keep a sense of proportion and know what is important. Demand scientific proof when it exists and base your treatment on scientific principles. The treatments of surgery, radiation, chemotherapy, and hormonal therapy have been scientifically tested in tens of thousands of breast cancer patients with consistent proven results.

Your first priority is to get well and stay well. If you don't have a choice and you need a mastectomy, then get one and look at the reconstruction options. Don't let the inconvenience or side effects of chemotherapy prevent you from receiving treatment if that is what you need. No one wants to lose her hair and feel poorly for four to six months, but you will recover and life should return to normal. However, relapsing metastatic breast cancer will change your life forever, so don't trade off cure rates against temporary side effects. Know what your priorities are and follow through on them.

It's normal to be fearful and upset at times. Rely on your medical team, friends, and family to help you get through this. Remember that you aren't alone. In 2004, there were 275,000 other people like you with a newly diagnosed breast cancer. Join a breast cancer support group. Rally your emotions and your determination. Fight your cancer and get well. Best wishes and good luck.

Appendix

GUIDE TO ONLINE BREAST CANCER RESOURCES

For information about breast cancer
American Cancer Society
www.cancer.org

BreastCancer.org
www.breastcancer.org

Living With It
www.livingwithit.org

National Cancer Institute
www.nci.nih.gov

National Women's Health Information Center
www.4woman.gov

People Living with Cancer
www.plwc.org

Susan G. Komen Foundation
www.breastcancerinfo.org

For information about fertility
Fertile Hope
www.fertilehope.org

For emotional support
CancerCare
www.cancercare.org

Cancervive
www.cancervive.org

FORCE, for BRCA positive women
www.facingourrisk.org

Friends in Need
www.friendsinneed.com

Gilda's Club
www.gildasclub.org

Lymphedema Network
www.lymphnet.org

Sister's Network, for African-American women
www.sistersnetworkinc.org

The Wellness Community
www.thewellnesscommunity.org

Y-ME National Breast Cancer Organization
www.y-me.org

Young Survival Coalition, for younger women
www.youngsurvival.org

Advocacy groups for policy issues
National Asian Women's Health Organization
www.nawho.org

National Breast Cancer Coalition
www.stopbreastcancer.org

National Coalition for Cancer Survivorship
www.canceradvocacy.org

National Women's Health Network
www.nwhn.org

Supporting breast cancer research
The Breast Cancer Research Foundation
www.bcrfcure.org

The Susan G. Komen Breast Cancer Foundation
www.breastcancerinfo.com

Glossary

Abraxane: A new intravenous chemotherapy that is a modification of Taxol and is currently only approved for use in advanced or metastatic breast cancer.

ADH: Atypical ductal hyperplasia. A condition of abnormal breast ducts that can only be diagnosed by biopsy and leads to a higher risk of breast cancer in the breast containing the abnormality.

adjuvant chemotherapy: The use of chemotherapy shortly following surgery to reduce breast cancer recurrence throughout the body.

Adriamycin: A commonly used intravenous chemotherapy for breast cancer from the class of drugs called anthracyclines.

alopecia: The medical term for hair loss.

Aloxi: A long active antinausea medication in the class called 5HT3 agonists that is given intravenously prior to chemotherapy treatments.

anemia: The condition of having a low red blood cell count that results in fatigue.

angiogenesis: The process of growing blood vessels. Cancers need this in order to obtain nutrition for growth.

antibiotic: Medications that fight bacterial infections. Medications that fight viral infections are called antivirals.

antiemetic: The medical term for any antinausea medication.

Anzimet: An antinausea medication in the class of 5HT3 agonists that can be taken by mouth or given intravenously.

Aranesp: A medication given by subcutaneous injection every two to three weeks that is used to correct chemotherapy caused anemia. This is essentially long acting Procrit.

areola: The darker and slightly raised area around the nipple.

Arimidex: The brand name for anastrozole, a hormonal treatment in pill form from the class of drugs called aromatase inhibitors. It is used in receptor positive postmenopausal patients only.

Aromasin: The brand name for exemestane, a hormonal treatment in pill form from the class of drugs called aromatase inhibitors. Used in receptor positive postmenopausal patients only.

aromatase inhibitor: A class of drugs in pill form used as hormonal therapy for breast cancer in postmenopausal patients who are hormone receptor positive. Aromatase inhibitors act to lower estrogen levels only in postmenopausal women. Drugs in the class are Arimidex, Femara, and Aromasin.

Avastin: A targeted therapy given intravenously that prevents blood vessel formation in cancer, thereby choking the cancer and causing it to shrink. Avastin is in a class of drugs called angiogenesis inhibitors.

axillary lymph node dissection: Surgery performed under the armpit to analyse whether or not the cancer has gone into lymph nodes.

benign: The medical term for not cancer.

bisphosphonates: A class of drugs that harden bone and reduce the ability of cancer to damage it. Intravenous drugs in this class are Aredia and Zometa. Oral drugs in the class are Fosamax and Actonel.

bone marrow: The center of hollow bones where blood elements are made.

bone marrow analysis: A test in which bone marrow is removed from the back of the pelvic bone to look for involvement by cancer or to assess how blood is being made.

bone marrow transplant: A technique for delivering very high doses of chemotherapy and/or radiation therapy. The bone marrow is removed before treatment to protect it from damage and then re-infused to allow normal blood production.

bone scan: A nuclear medicine test to assess bone activity that sometimes can indicate spread of cancer into bones. A radioactive substance is injected intravenously, followed by a scan several hours later.

BRCA: A genetic blood test for breast cancer susceptibility gene for certain forms of inherited breast cancer.

cardiomyopathy: Weakening of the heart muscle so that it can't pump blood well.

chemotherapy: Drugs that are taken either by mouth or, more commonly, intravenously that damage cancer by preventing DNA replication and cell division.

clinical trials: Experimental studies conducted scientifically to test the effectiveness of a treatment or intervention.

Compazine: A commonly used antinausea pill. It is also available as a suppository.

CT scan: A computer generated X-ray that permits visualization of internal body structures. Typically, contrast material is given by mouth and intravenously to highlight internal organs.

Cytoxan: The brand name for cyclophosphamide. a commonly used chemotherapy. It can be taken by pill or be given intravenously.

DCIS: An abbreviation for ductal carcinoma in situ, a noninvasive form of breast cancer.

Decadron: The brand name of dexamethasone, a steroid commonly used as an antinausea medication and frequently given by intravenous injection prior to receiving chemotherapy. It is also used as a premedication for Taxol and Taxotere.

Depolupron: A medication given by intramuscular injection that stops the production of estrogen by the ovaries. This medication can temporarily change menopause status from premenopause to postmenopause.

DIEP flap: A type of tissue reconstruction using skin and fat, usually from the abdomen, in which the tissue is completely freed, without blood supply from the body, prior to its use for reconstructive purposes.

dose-dense chemotherapy: A technique of giving chemotherapy in which the treatments are compressed and given more frequently.

ductal lavage: A diagnostic technique in which a small tube is inserted into a breast duct in the nipple to test for the presence of cancer cells.

ductogram: A diagnositic test in which a small tube is inserted into a breast duct in the nipple and contrast is injected while X-rays are taken.

Ellence: The brand name for epirubicin, a commonly used intravenous chemotherapy drug in the class called anthracyclines.

Emend: An antinausea medication that is given in pill form, starting before chemotherapy is administered. It affects a newly identified group of receptors called NK1 and is helpful in reducing delayed nausea.

Epirubicin: The chemical name for Ellence, a commonly used chemotherapy in the class of drugs called anthracyclines.

ER: Abbreviation for estrogen receptor.

Estring: A medication providing low dose estrogen in the vagina via a small ring placed within the vagina and replaced every three months.

estrogen: A female hormone that stimulates breast development and can encourage growth of some breast cancer cells; estrogen declines as a woman becomes menopausal.

estrogen receptor: The binding site of estrogen on breast cancer cells, which indicates an ability of the cancer to be affected by changes in hormone levels.

extravasation: Leakage from the vein during a chemotherapy infusion. This is a problem with some chemotherapy drugs that are very irritating to the skin.

Evista: The brand name for raloxifen, a hormonal drug in pill form with breast cancer activity, from the class of drugs called SERMs. Evista blocks estrogen and progesterone receptors.

Fareston: A hormonal therapy in pill form with Tamoxifen-like activity, a SERM. Fareston blocks estrogen and progesterone receptors.

Faslodex: A hormonal therapy for receptor positive metastatic breast cancer given by intramuscular injection monthly. Faslodex degrades estrogen receptors.

Femara: The brand name for letrozole, a hormonal therapy in pill form in the class of aromatase inhibitors, used for receptor positive postmenopausal patients only.

G-CSF: An abbreviation often used for Neupogen, a drug given sub-cutaneously on a daily basis to raise white blood cell counts.

Gemzar: The brand name for gemcitabine, a chemotherapy drug given by intravenous injection and used for metastatic breast cancer.

gene microarray: A technology for analyzing genetic material from a biopsy sample.

GM-CSF: An abbreviation often used for Leukine, a drug given sub-cutaneously on a daily basis to raise white blood cell counts.

granulocytes: Also called neutrophils. One type of white blood cells that functions to fight bacterial infections. Granulocytes keep blood from becoming infected.

Her2: A non-inherited genetic abnormality occurring in some breast cancers that makes the cancer susceptible to Herceptin. Her2 is tested on the biopsy specimen.

Herceptin: A targeted monoclonal antibody treatment given intravenously for patients who have Her2 mutations.

hormonal therapy: Any manipulation of hormone status or function in the treatment of cancer.

infiltrating ductal carcinoma: Also known as invasive ductal carcinoma. This is the most common type of invasive breast cancer.

inflammatory breast cancer: An aggressive form of invasive breast cancer that causes redness and swelling of the breast.

intravenous: Abbreviated as IV, injection of medications into the vein.

Ki-67: A test performed on biopsied breast cancer cells that measures the potential growth rate of a cancer. A higher number indicates a faster growing cancer.

Kytril: An antinausea medication in the class of 5HT3 agonists that can be given in pill or intravenous form.

LCIS: An abbreviation for lobular carcinoma in situ. This abnormality increases breast cancer risk in both breasts, not just the breast containing LCIS.

Leukine: A medication given by subcutaneous injection daily to raise white blood cell counts.

lobular carcinoma: A type of invasive breast cancer sometimes referred to as invasive lobular carcinoma.

lobular carcinoma in situ (LCIS): A noninvasive type of breast cancer abbreviated as LCIS.

lumpectomy: the surgical technique of removing a breast cancer by removing only the part of the breast containing the cancer, leaving the remainder of the breast intact.

lymphedema: A condition in which the arm and hand are swollen as a consequence of damage to the lymphatic system.

mammogram: An X-ray to image breast tissue.

Mammosite: A technique of limited or partial radiation therapy of the breast.

malignant.: The medical term for something that is cancer.

mastectomy: A surgical technique in which the entire breast is removed.

Megace: The brand name of a hormonal therapy in pill form that is progesterone based.

metastasis: A term used to describe a situation in which cancer has spread. In the case of breast cancer, the term is used when cancer has spread to areas outside of the breast and lymph nodes of the armpit.

modified radical mastectomy: A surgical technique in which the entire breast and many lymph nodes within the armpit are removed.

MRI: An abbreviation for magnetic resonance imaging, a computerized image created using electromagnetic fields rather than X-rays.

nausea: The sensation of needing to vomit.

neoadjuvant chemotherapy: Preoperative chemotherapy, the use of chemotherapy before surgery, often used to reduce the size of the breast cancer before the operation while at the same time reducing relapse rates throughout the body.

Neulasta: The long acting form of Neupogen given subcutaneously to raise white blood cell counts.

Neumega: A drug injected subcutaneously on a daily basis to raise platelet counts.

Neupogen: A drug injected subcutaneously on a daily basis to raise white blood cell counts.

neutrophils: Also called granulocytes. A type of white blood cell that fights bacterial infections and keeps blood from becoming infected.

Oncotype DX: A test of gene function used to try to predict breast cancer behavior and relapse risk. The test is performed on biopsy material.

Paclitaxel: The chemical name for Taxol, a commonly used intravenous chemotherapy in the class of drugs called taxanes.

Paget's disease: A term for DCIS within the nipple.

Pamidronate: The chemical name for Aredia, an intravenous drug given to strengthen bones.

partial mastectomy: More commonly referred to as a lumpectomy.

PET scan: A nuclear medicine test used to try determine cancer location within the body based on different rates of blood sugar (glucose) use by cancer versus normal tissues.

phytoestrogens: Plant substances that have estrogen-like activity.

placebo: A substance containing no medicine. It may be given for psychological effect. Placebos are sometimes given during clinical trials to disguise whether or not a patient is receiving the experimental drug being tested.

platelets: A blood component that prevents bleeding.

port: A device used for intravenous access.

postmenopausal: The state of being in menopause in which menstrual periods have ceased and estrogen levels are low.

PR: An abbreviation for progesterone receptor.

Procrit: A medication given subcutaneously on a weekly basis to raise red blood cell counts.

progesterone receptor: The binding site of progestorone on breast cancer cells, which indicates the ability of the cancer to be affected by changes in hormone levels.

proteomics: Tests of protein function used to predict cancer behavior, response to treatment, and recurrence risk.

radiation therapy: The technique of using high energy X-ray to destroy cancer.

radical mastectomy: a surgery that is no longer used in which the entire breast, chest muscles, and lymph nodes were removed.

segmental mastectomy: The technical term for a lumpectomy in which only the portion of the breast containing cancer is removed.

sentinel node biopsy: A surgical technique in which only limited numbers of lymph nodes are removed from the armpit to detect whether breast cancer spread has occurred. A blue dye and a radio-active tracer are used to locate the sentinel nodes.

skin-sparing mastectomy: the surgical technique of performing a mastectomy without completely removing the skin of the breast to enhance reconstruction of the breast.

SERM: An abbreviation for selective estrogen receptor modulators, a class of hormonal therapy that includes Tamoxifen, Fareston, and Evista.

SSRI: An abbreviation for a class of antidepressant medications that affect the neurotransmitter serotonin, selective serotonin reuptake inhibitor.

subcutaneous: Abbreviated SQ, and meaning injection of medication under the skin.

Tamoxifen: A hormonal treatment in pill form in a class of drugs called SERMs. Tamoxifen blocks estrogen and progesterone receptors. The brand name is Nolvadex.

Taxol: The brand name for paclitaxel, a chemotherapy in the class of drugs called taxanes.

TMN: The staging system for cancers including breast cancer. The system takes into account the size of the cancer, lymph node involvement, and whether or not metastases are present.

TRAM reconstruction: A technique of breast reconstruction using abdominal skin, fat, and muscle with the blood supply intact.

tumor markers: Blood tests that are used to measure the presence or absence of cancer.

ultrasound: An imaging technique in which sound waves are used to detect abnormalities.

Vagifem: An estrogen suppository that delivers small amounts of estrogen to the vagina.

Xeloda: The brand name for capcitabine, a chemotherapy pill used for treating metastatic breast cancer.

Zofran: An 5HT3 antinausea medication available in pill and intravenous form, as well as in a sublingual formulation for dissolving under the tongue.

Zoladex: A medication given intramuscularly to reduce estrogen production from the ovaries.

Zometa: The brand name for zoledronate, an intravenous medication given monthly to strengthen the bones and reduce cancer damage.

Acknowledgments

T HIS BOOK WAS written at the urging of Kathy Calderon, NP, a skilled and compassionate breast cancer support group leader in Redondo Beach, California. Frustrated by the lack of detailed and yet understandable information about their illness, she and her patients wanted a comprehensive breast cancer book specific enough to help most women address their individual circumstances while answering the questions that were foremost on their minds. *Breast Cancer: Real Questions, Real Answers* was formulated chapter by chapter from questions and answers reviewed by Kathy and members of her breast cancer support group, all of whom I thank for their indispensable contribution.

Each chapter includes vignettes of actual patients to illustrate and highlight important points. The patients' names and circumstances have been altered to protect their privacy.

The initial draft was reviewed by leading cancer specialists to ensure that the information in the book is comprehensive and accurate. I want to acknowledge the contributions of Dr. George Canellos, Dr. Linnea Chap, Dr. Douglas Blayney, Dr. Cliff Hudis, and in particular Dr.

Peter Ravdin who dissected the first draft sentence by sentence, providing me with excellent suggestions as well as appreciated criticism.

The illustrations and tables were created by Dr. Eric Glassy, a leading pathologist and a talented medical illustrator. Dr. Glassy's vision and expertise were invaluable, and from the beginning gave me a clear view of what the final book would become. A huge debt of gratitude is owed to Dr. Oi-Lin Chen of Sunrider International for her very generous donation of copies for breast cancer patients. Many thanks to my friend and colleague, Dr. John Glaspy, and my friend and mentor, Dr. Frank Stockdale, for their contributions to the book, and more importantly for their steadfast support over many years. I want to acknowledge with gratitude and affection my professor and chairman, Dr. Saul Rosenberg, for teaching me how to care for cancer patients. My father, a poet and professor, taught me how to write. I lovingly thank him for that and also for his help with the many drafts as the book developed. *Breast Cancer: Real Questions, Real Answers* would never have been published without the efforts of my brother Kip, a professor and author, who has been my steady guide through the arcane world of publishing.

A big hug of appreciation goes to my friends and staff at Cancer Care Associates, and to Drs. Nora Ku and Mark Pegram for their friendship and support.

Lastly, this would not have been possible without the tremendous love and encouragement of my family, especially my wonderful black belt computer wiz son, Spencer, and my beautiful wife, Suzy.

Index

NOTE: Page numbers in *italics* indicate an illustration or chart.